DETOX YOURSELF

The Secret to Freeing Your Mind and
Creating a Healthy Life

R.L. Malpica

ISBN: 979-8-9994152-0-2

Published by Nature Over Everything Publishing

This book is intended for informational purposes only and does not constitute medical advice.

First edition, 2025

Printed in the United States of America

Dedicated to all of humanity. The ripple effect of becoming the best version of yourself will make this world a better place.

Acknowledgments

First and foremost, I want to acknowledge my wife, Ryan — the real one behind all of this. Your support, your belief in me, and your love have fueled everything I've created. You've always been my biggest fan, my challenger when I needed it, and the most consistent source of inspiration in my life. I truly wouldn't be who I am or be doing any of this without you.

To my daughter Dom — you've inspired me more than you probably know. Watching you grow into your own, seeing you chase your path, it's motivated me to keep becoming a better man. You've helped shape me in ways I'll always be grateful for.

To my daughter Nadia — you are a driving force in my life. Every day I wake up thinking about the legacy I'm building for you — one that carries truth, strength, and freedom. I hope this book becomes something you can grow with, something that plants values deep and helps break the cycles we weren't meant to carry.

To my daughter June — thank you for challenging me in the best ways. You've helped me realize how important it is to lay down a solid foundation, one you can build on as you walk your own journey through life.

Everything I write is for you girls — so you can see the world for what it really is, question everything, live intentionally, and create a life rooted in real health and truth.

To my mom — thank you for always making me believe I could do anything in this life. That mindset is everything.

To my brother Lou — thank you for all the energy and love you've poured into my life, don't know where I'd be without it bro. To my brother Nabil — thank you for the creative inspiration and always sharing love with your big brother. You've sparked a lot of what lives in these pages. To my Uncle Vince — you're always there and always supporting with love, can't tell you how much that means to me. To my sister Bernie — thank you for your unwavering love and support. And to my cousin Kim — thank you for always showing love, no matter what. Your support and energy are always felt.

To my circle of brothers — Eric, Darko, Ryan, Matt, and Crane — y'all have always been real ones. You've pushed me, motivated me, held me accountable, and most importantly, you've just been there. I appreciate you more than words can capture.

To Dr. Robert Morse — your teachings laid the foundation for everything I talk about in this book. The way you blend the spiritual with the physical is something I strive for in my own voice. Your work, your school, your approach — it all shaped my understanding of healing and helped me reconnect with what's real. I hope to carry that forward in my own way.

To Lauren Farris — thank you for being a mentor and guiding light. Your Facebook group, *Terrain Model Refutes Germ Theory*, shifted the entire direction of my family's life. You showed up at just the right time

— during one of the most challenging periods — and gave me clarity that led to this book even existing. I've learned so much from you, and I'm forever grateful.

To Yah'ki — thank you for showing me the deeper understanding of how the body works and how to present that knowledge with clarity. You've helped shape not just what I teach but how I teach.

To Dr. Douglas Graham — your book *The 80/10/10 Diet* flipped my understanding of food upside down and became a massive pillar of my philosophy. Thank you for that paradigm shift.

To my *Escape Within* family — you already know. The way you support me in everything I do is unmatched. You push me to step out of my comfort zone and into my role as a lightworker, and I'm better because of all of you.

And lastly — to myself.
Thank you for staying true, for continuing to grow in a world that often wants to keep you small. For moving through trauma, for staying grounded in your purpose, for showing up every day and doing the work. You've endured, evolved, and chosen the light, over and over again. I see you, and I'm proud of you.

I know there are people I've missed — please know I feel your love. If you're reading this and you've played any role in my life, you're a part of this story, and I appreciate you deeply.

Introduction

It's funny how an idea can create its own energy and manifest into something completely different than the original thought. I wanted to write a book about a philosophy that I created along my own personal journey of salvation. Throughout my journey from a lost soul traveling across this earthly plane to an awakened beacon of light, I experienced a very succinct transformation that formulated the man I am today. I called it my path to enlightenment which included the process of breaking my conditioning, creating a healthy terrain, obtaining oneness and then exploring spirituality.

The outline of the book was set. It was going to be four parts diving into each aspect of the four pillars. So, what happened? As is common in life, the universe had other plans. At the time of the idea's birth, I was a freethinking light-working truth-seeker. While I still consider myself all of the aforementioned labels, my true passion changed in 2020.

On March 11, 2020, the World Health Organization declared Covid-19 a pandemic. I remember my wife and I contemplating how we were going to operate moving forward. We were like most of the population, not sure who to believe, but we knew what was coming. Being a truth seeker, I took in all the information with a grain of salt. My years of awakening helped me quickly realize that what was transpiring before our eyes was nothing more than a theatrical performance.

My focus quickly shifted to understanding the nuances of the human body. If the country I live in, and in some cases the state I live in, was going to mandate health related guidelines, I was going to know everything I could about health. Through my exploration, I stumbled upon a Facebook group called *Terrain model refutes germ theory* which showed me a completely different way to look at our diet. A natural way. The conversations within this group immediately resonated with my overall view of health. Lauren Farris, the admin of the group and Natural Hygienist, was like a mentor to me and provided such detailed information of how the body works. I even had her on my podcast a couple times. It was a like another awakening! I started reading books, watching documentaries, listening to natural health related podcasts and most importantly, implementing the natural health concepts into my life.

All of a sudden, it became my life. My diet changed. My view of germs changed... and most importantly, my health changed. I lost roughly 30lbs and eliminated previous ailments including battles with eczema, irritable bowel syndrome and chronic headaches. My body was being cured, not treated. With that, my book changed. Not because I don't believe in my concepts anymore, but because my experience changed. Oneness is a personal experience that cannot be encapsulated in a book by somebody else. Yes, I could have written a book about my personal oneness experience and it may have resonated with people, but that's what podcasts are for. Yes, I could have shared all of my amazing spiritual experiences from mystical meditations, mind-blowing reiki sessions and astral projections, but that's my journey, not yours.

I chose to focus on the two aspects that I'm not only most passionate about, but I feel will truly transform your life so you CAN obtain true oneness and free your mind to truly explore all the amazing features this universe provides.

My intention for this book is to open your eyes to a reality that you may not have known existed. Some of the information may be familiar, but my goal is to help you understand the impact.

This is not a self-help book, it's a wake-up call. I chose to keep this book in the same vein as my approach to understanding life; Simple. You won't find too much medical jargon or complex verbiage because honestly, it's not needed. Complicated words and scientific terminology has its place, but it's mostly used to confuse the observer. As you'll learn throughout this book, that is by design.

Read pretty much any medical journal, article or reference book and you'll see exactly what I'm talking about. By the time you get a paragraph or two in, your head will start to hurt. Law books and legislature are the same way. Those periodicals are industry, or should I say, system specific. They're written in a different language on purpose. The more we, as a people, understand... the more we question. The more we question, the more we start to realize that the answers don't make sense.

You may be asking, *what does this have to do with creating a healthier life?* The answer is... everything.

Creating a healthy life can be very simple, but the systems that have been put in place, most likely before you were ever born, make it difficult.

My entire premise behind this book is to help you see what's been hidden in plain sight. The world as you know it is not set up to see you succeed or for you to live a healthy fulfilling life. Nor is it set up for you to have the opportunity to uncover that unfortunate truth.

This is not a health book. There are plenty of natural health books that are amazing at what they do. As you'll see, I quote some incredible health related works like *The Detox Miracle Sourcebook* by Robert Morse, N.D., *The 80/10/10 Diet* by Dr. Douglas N. Graham and *What Really Makes You Ill? - Why Everything You Thought You Knew About Disease is Wrong* by Dawn Lester and David Parker. These are very substantial sources that have been building blocks for my own personal philosophies on health.

When it comes to making choices in life, our job is never to follow, but to gather all of the information at our disposal and make a conscious decision. I implore you to do the same after reading this book. Some of my ideas may trigger you, but understand that everything I share in the following pages is coming from a place of love. We're all a part of a collective consciousness and all play a pivotal role in the manifestation of our world around us.

We are a product of our environment, so if our environment is toxic, then guess what we become? So how do we change our environment? How do we control the circumstances that affect our life on a daily basis? How do we change our inner and outer terrain to promote vitality? How do we become the best version of ourselves? It starts with detoxing yourself... but before you can detox yourself, you have to understand how you've been intoxicated.

Part One
Freeing Your Mind

Break Your Conditioning

"We're addicted to our beliefs; we're addicted to the emotions of our past. We see our beliefs as truths, not ideas that we can change... and many of these things are having a negative impact on our health and happiness." - Dr. Joe Dispenza

I often use the phrase "all by design" when referring to happenings of everyday society. One of the major issues with the individual of today, is that we take the most basic core foundation of our being for granted; the mind. It's the easiest functional part of our body to overlook because it doesn't have a physical function like the rest of our body. That's why the majority of people can be brainwashed, conditioned and programmed without even knowing it. So, if you take a deep look at society, you'll be able to see that your reality is merely a projection of your programming. It's all by design.

From the commercials you see on television subliminally depositing messages into your subconscious to the idealism of beauty through a shallow depiction of vanity, it's all by design. The design has been, and always will be, to control you. The easiest way to control you is to manipulate your emotions based on root level programming. We've all been conditioned since the moment we were born. From the roots. This isn't your fault, remember, it's all by design. A design that was concocted generations ago by low-level consciousness and dark entities who share a lack of humanity and feed off of our struggles.

But this isn't about them... this is about you.

You're probably asking yourself what does breaking my conditioning have to do with my health? The truth is, conditioning is the reason you see health the way it is today in the first place. My goal is to help you break your conditioning so you can start with a clean slate, absorb the information, and be able to make a conscious decision on what's best for you and your family.

By understanding and acknowledging that you've been conditioned, it enables you to open your mind and realize that some of the most fundamental aspects of health that you've been taught are completely wrong. I want to give you an overall picture of how the world works and how conditioning works and how it's a part of every single element of your life. From there, you'll be able to see how it's all connected.

How do you break years of conditioning? Years of brainwashing? Years of programming? Is it possible to remove decades of misinformation and indoctrination from your memory? The short answer is yes, but it starts with one of the most fundamental concepts of life; acknowledgement.

Now look, no one wants to admit that they've been conditioned or programmed. It's not like it's something to brag about and while humbleness is a feat that a good majority of us possess, I'd venture to say more people suffer from the ego-driven personality traits of stubbornness and pride.

Acknowledgment is where it starts.

About eight years ago, I finally acknowledged that I was heavily conditioned. It took a lot for me to come to terms with it, but once I did, there was no turning back. An entire new world was opened and the possibilities seemed endless! Honestly, it was tough to get there... tough to let go of everything I had been taught... and even tougher realizing that the world as I knew it, was a lie.

My heaviest form of conditioning stemmed from one of the most powerful entities on the planet and where I feel the origins of programming started; religion.

Throughout my life, my religious activity and interest had wavered back and forth. Being of Hispanic descent, it's no surprise that my family practiced the Catholic religion. I was baptized Catholic. Both my older brother and mother went to Catholic school. Crosses. Rosaries. Traditions. Growing up, this was just a part of life. Not a choice, but reality. When you're told something as a child, especially from your parents, it resonates on a deep level. Your parents are your world... and ultimately, the biggest influence in your life. There's no challenging those ideas. It just is what it is. If you grow up in America, there's a really good chance that you'll be exposed, conditioned and indoctrinated by some form of Christianity. If not Christianity, then possibly Islam, Judaism or another form of organized religion.

I consider religion the origin of programming because of the power in which it possesses. It's the ultimate tool to control. By using a higher being or beings as the foundation of law mixed with the power of fear, religion has and continues to literally control the lives of billions. When you take a deep look at Christianity, the most dominant religion of the past 2000 years, you'll get a clear picture of the power behind conditioning. Christian influences are spread throughout society, from not being able to buy liquor on Sunday in some states to the on-going legislative discrimination against the LGBT community. How about gender discrimination, roles and pay gap? All of this stems from Christianity in America. If you need further proof of Christianity as a brainwashing tool, look no further than the Atlantic Slave Trade. Africans were forced to practice the religion with the idealism of white supremacy supported by the doctrine.

"Servants, be obedient to them that are your masters according to the flesh, with fear and trembling, in singleness of your heart, as unto Christ; not with eye-service, as men-pleasers; but as the servants of Christ, doing the will of God from the heart; with good will doing service, as to the Lord, and not to men: knowing that whatsoever good thing any man doeth, the same shall he receive of the Lord, whether he be bond or free." - Ephesians VI 5-7

Books such as *How To Make a Negro Christian* and *The Religious Instruction of the Negroes in the United States* go into explicit detail about the conditioning used to indoctrinate an entire race of people.

By the time I was 33 years old, Christianity was so embedded into my being, that the thought of a world outside of the Christian faith seemed outrageous. I was extremely conditioned.

One of my best friends and someone I consider a brother, Eric Deshun Edwards, became a major culprit to the acknowledgment of my conditioning. Along with being one of my closest friends, he was also my barber. A couple times a month, I'd head to his shop for a quick cut and deep conversation. Topics spanned from sports to video games to relationships, but once religion was brought up, the exchanges became a bit more passionate. Eric had already come to the conclusion that Christianity, and all religions for that matter, were just another form of indoctrination. At the time, I was suffering from a psychological disorder known as cognitive dissonance. It didn't matter what he said, how much sense he was making or the lack of proof I could provide to support my beliefs, at the end of the day, I didn't want to acknowledge it because it would shatter a part of my life that I'd always thought was true.

It took a major moment in my daughter's life to push me over the edge.

I had Dom when I was 17 years old. I was just a young dumb kid with zero self-esteem on the verge of bringing life into the world. It forced me to grow up fast and naturally, and I leaned on traditional values to raise my little girl. At the time, it felt right. I was very adamant about her doing well in school, following my somewhat strict rules and abiding by the conformity of society.

When she was a junior in high school, I found out she had been smoking weed with some of her friends. I pulled her out of school, drove her to an empty parking lot and stopped the car.

"There something you want to tell me?" I asked rhetorically.

"Umm... no," she responded obliviously.

She had no idea that I knew about the weed. I had no idea there was something else.

Just like the way I was brought up, I raised Dom in the Christian faith. Baptized her when she was ten. Church most Sundays. We hadn't had many deep talks regarding Christianity, but she knew the doctrine. And anyone who knows the doctrine, understands the Christian stance on homosexuality, so when she came out and told her mother and I that she was bisexual, it was the first time my faith had been truly challenged.

I was brainwashed, but the moment I found out about Dom and her sexuality, something happened. It was like a vail was pulled from over my eyes and I began to question everything I had ever been taught. Not that I had anything against her coming out, I was just heavily conditioned to look at it from a Christian perspective. From that moment on, I started heavily researching Christianity from non-Christian sources. Everything Eric was saying was true... I was just too blind to see it.

That's why acknowledgement is so difficult for people. It's not as much the admitting you're wrong, it's more about the shame that comes with being fooled. Being able to look into the mirror and admit to yourself that you were wrong is a tough pill to swallow for most individuals. It's like realizing you're a robot who's been programmed to act the way you do. Everything from the way you talk, react, feel... almost as if your entire identity was predetermined.

There are three categories of people... the awakened, those on the path to becoming awakened and those who don't even realize they are asleep. We are all healing in our own ways, even those in the latter category... but remember, words are powerless on deaf ears. The conditioning of society is strong... so strong that those who are asleep are more concerned about the comfortability of their bed instead of focusing on the time they need to wake up in the morning... they get so comfortable, that once that alarm starts ringing, their first, second and third response is to push the snooze button. They don't want to wake up. Why would they? They're relaxed... secure in their top of the line sleep number bed... where they don't have to deal with the inconvenient truth, the uncomfortable realities of society or the blatant downfall of humanity. Giving up those accommodations constitutes a change in mindset both mentally and spiritually. That's work... sacrifice... something most are unwilling to give for the betterment of our collective consciousness. Why, you ask? Because most people focus on the transformation, not the transformed.

Luckily for you, you've already taken the first step to changing your life. You're on the path to breaking free of the conditioning that's been thrust upon you from the moment you were born. But understand, this journey is work. Every day you'll be challenged by a conditioned society who have yet to realize they are operating under a systemic program. Work will challenge you. The news will challenge you. Social media will challenge you. Your friends will challenge you. Family will challenge you.

One of the most challenging aspects of breaking your conditioning is living in a world where the majority of people don't see things the way you do. Don't allow the masses to stunt your growth. This is all a part of the process. Remember, most people operate with a hive mind and usually submit to a group think mentality. It's okay to go against the grain if it aligns with your values.

You are on your own journey towards a healthier and more prosperous life. Sometimes it can be a lonely journey, but rest assured, there should be no compromise when it comes to becoming the best version of yourself.

In the beginning...

"Before you heal someone, ask them if they are willing to give up the things that made them sick." - Hippocrates

Now, I'm no physician, but this quote relates to all aspects of life. Are you willing to give up life as you know it? As you see it? As you feel it?

It's a very deep question that most may answer superficially, but when it comes down to the actual transformation, the question can become a daily battle. Most people think a spiritual awakening is an immediate metamorphosis accompanied by some metaphysical experience that changes one's outlook on life forever. While I have heard of these types of experiences, they are far from the norm when you first get on the path. It's about work... inner work.

Like I said earlier, conditioning is generational. We are merely products of our parents, family, environment and society. You are born into conditioning. And for the first eighteen-years of your life, you're treated like a product more than an actual human being. I allude to the first eighteen years only because you're considered a dependent by society. Most people are conditioned and stay conditioned their entire life. As you'll see, the brainwashing, indoctrination and conditioning come from all aspects of your life. Society has built-in systems that were created to mold you into a submissive modern-day slave of civilization.

Remember, the first step towards creating a healthy life is breaking your conditioning, but even before that, you have to acknowledge that you've been conditioned in the first place. You have to acknowledge the intoxication. And to acknowledge something, you have to be convinced. But just like my experience with Eric, you're going to have to convince yourself. My job is to make you think... open your mind... consider the possibilities... and most importantly, question everything.

So where does it begin? Let's take a look at the typical journey through life in today's society.

The moment a child is born, they're immediately interjected into the medical system. I'll spend more time breaking down the medical and health care system in the next section, but for now, let's touch on the surface. A newborn is given a vitamin K and a Hepatitis B vaccine at birth. If you're asking how this pertains to conditioning, the answer can vary based on your stance towards vaccines. Once again, I will dive deeper into vaccines in the next chapter. Let's start by looking at things logically. The birthing process is an extremely traumatic event for a baby. Why anyone would want to inject a newborn with toxic chemicals after such an event is beyond me, but when you look at vaccines in their totality, you quickly realize that it's just the beginning of a designed plan. Remember, it's all by design.

The problem is that most parents don't question their doctors. This is where the generational conditioning comes into play. Older generations were taught to never question authoritative figures like doctors. They were raised under the programming that doctors are not to be questioned. You feel sick, go to the doctor and accept whatever diagnosis is given. This filters right into the moment of birth. The doctor doesn't ask the parents whether or not they want to vaccinate their child at birth, they just do it. Status quo.

Yes, parents can request to not have their child vaccinated at birth but the conditioning is so strong, that it rarely happens.

Why? Simple... because parents are conditioned to have faith in their doctors and the health care system with no resistance.

Question a doctor? Why would anyone question a doctor?

Because if you can't trust everything, you have to question everything. Even doctors. You have to understand that doctors received their medical license, knowledge and training from institutions that are a part of a system. The medical system. That system has parameters that were created with more than the well-being of society as its motivation. By no means am I saying that doctors are incompetent, I'm just pointing out the facts. Doctors can be questioned too. They are not an authority figure... and it's you and your family's body. There are plenty of physicians that think outside of the box and take a more alternative approach to healing, and if you search hard enough, you'll find them. Unfortunately, the majority of doctors are conditioned as well.

For example, when my youngest daughter was born, we wanted to find a pediatrician that was pro-choice when it came to vaccines. Most pediatricians won't accept patients who don't vaccinate. All we wanted was a choice in the matter. We found a family clinic that claimed to be natural and alternative, but ended up leaving after a few visits. My whole point in this matter is that when we're talking about the health and wellness of our most prized possessions, our children, we should take the time and effort to ensure they are getting the best care possible. Not what the government tells us, but what we've concluded after our own personal research.

Now back to the vaccines and the designed plan. Have you ever asked yourself why would a less than a day-old newborn baby need a Hepatitis B vaccine?

Per *CDC.gov*, Hepatitis B is spread when blood, semen, or other body fluids from a person infected with the virus enters the body of someone who is not infected. This can happen through sexual contact; sharing needles, syringes, or other drug-injection equipment; or from mother to baby at birth.

Read that again and ask yourself why a newborn baby would need this vaccine at birth or any time before his/her teenage years, if at all. Even the misleading "from mother to baby at birth" argument is moot considering vaccines are supposedly given to prevent disease, not cure it.

It doesn't stop there... no, it's just getting started.

By the time you were 12 months old, you were vaccinated over thirty times. While this speaks more to your parent's conditioning than yours, it's the genesis of your programming. Remember, your parents were the biggest influence in your life. Your values, traditions, morals and beliefs stem from your upbringing.

The whole vaccination debate is a completely different conversation. My point is centered on the indoctrination of society regarding vaccinations. People should be informed, aware and not ridiculed for their personal choices. We're talking about unnatural toxic chemicals being put into children's bodies at the early stages of development. It's impossible to know the true long-term effects of vaccines or any medicine administered to kids because it's too difficult to conduct long term trials, not to mention the ethics of experimenting on children. There are too many outside factors that take place over a long span of time. But when we see major increases in cognitive disorders like Autism, ADHD and other intellectual disabilities, one can only question the possible underlying triggers.

As of 2017, the *CDC* estimated that about one in six, or about 17%, of children aged 3 through 17 years had one or more developmental disabilities. To put things into perspective, it was 13.8% as of 2008. Over the last 12 years, the prevalence of Autism increased by 289.5% and ADHD increased by 33%.

The amount of vaccines recommended for children has increased dramatically. Per childrenshealthdefense.org, in 1986, 12 vaccines were recommended for a child up to the age of 14. As of 2021, 49 vaccines were recommended.

These numbers do not equate to absolute causation of any disorder, but at the same time, they cannot be ignored. I am merely trying to open your mind to start asking questions. I do not advocate for vaccinations, but I highly recommend the book *The Vaccine-Friendly Plan* written by Paul Thomas M.D. and Jennifer Margulis Ph.D. if you decide to vaccinate your children.

We're already a part of the plan within minutes of our birth. Add in the registration for a social security number and a birth certificate, and we're officially members of the system.

Historian Jordan Maxwell says of birth certificates, "Birth certificates are a certificate of manifest... because you are a corporate owned item, a human resource."

Corporate OWNED item? A human RESOURCE?

Yes. We are a resource. We're born into an assembly line... or better yet a massive controlled herd. Let me continue.

The power of the media through endless propaganda may be the single most influential medium in society. Generations of people have been conditioned to welcome television and now social media as pillars of the family home. The results have been a dumbed down culture who follows trends, looks at vanity as validation and judgment as a means to credibility.

One way in which the media has had a profound effect on children and the future of our planet is food. The *CDC* reports that only 47% of babies born are breastfed exclusively at 3 months despite reduced risks of asthma, obesity, type 2 diabetes and other debilitating diseases. Why? Some mothers cannot produce, but others have been programmed to think that formula is sufficient. Some fall victim to generational ignorance. Tell me if you've heard this one before...

"Well, I wasn't breastfed and I turned out fine..."

Some mothers do not want to deal with the hassle.

Breastmilk is the most natural, organic and healthy form of food in nature. The fact that billion-dollar corporations like Nestle and Kraft use enticing advertising to manipulate the subconscious minds of parents is absolutely disturbing. Once again, the motive is never the betterment of the people.

In an article from The Guardian publication *How formula milk firms target mothers who can least afford it* — "Formula milk companies are continuing to use aggressive, clandestine and often illegal methods to target mothers in the poorest parts of the world to encourage them to choose powdered milk over breastfeeding..."

This form of conditioning continues throughout your life. Think about the commercials on television or in-between acts on your favorite streaming channels. Count how many times you see a commercial promoting breastfeeding or organic fruits and vegetables.

Multi-million-dollar advertising firms are hired by billion-dollar corporations to formulate a plan to hijack your subconscious mind. They pull countless amounts of data and separate their targets, the people, into different groups called demographics. Corporations also keep data on which products are successful with each specific demographic. The entire process is a microcosm of society. It's about control... being able to control their clientele. The more information they have, the more ammunition they can use to manipulate your emotions.

It doesn't stop at commercials. It's extremely prevalent in the entire entertainment industry. The public has been brainwashed to believe that the only way to be relevant and achieve self-worth is to acquire societal validation. This validation stems from pop culture and industry trends.

Have you ever stopped to ask yourself why you dress the way you do? Or why you want a specific car? Specific type of house? Have you ever taken a step back to dissect who you are?

Most individuals go through multiple serious relationships before finally finding someone they truly want to spend the rest of their life with. There are many different factors that come into play when it comes to love, but one of the biggest issues is conditioning. We've been programmed through television and the media to a superficial standard of beauty. We've also been brainwashed through patriarchy and chauvinistic traditions to believe in definitive gender roles. This generational cycle has not only affected relationships and marriages, it's also affected the self-worthiness and self-esteem of women.

We're all taught that blue is for boys and pink is for girls.

"Boys don't cry."

"Don't act like a girl."

Boys have to be tough and they can't be emotional. Then Disney movies and other forms of entertainment build this expectation of a fairy tale love that captures the imagination of the youth. This is all conditioning!

When kids are sent to school with other conditioned kids, it only exemplifies the programming and further instills the conditioning. Remember, a kid's ability to be influenced is at its highest point during childhood. After their parents, next in line is their associates. Their peers.

So, when kids go to school with other conditioned kids, that conditioning is validated. There's strength in numbers and when children are all brought up the same way, it lessens the urge for curiosity. In moments when there is a conflict in ideology, a child is usually told to dismiss it and not ask questions.

Which brings me to the education system. Now, I understand the importance of schooling and also, the difficulties in building a sustainable system to teach the youth. By no means am I discrediting all of the amazing teachers who dedicate their lives to the betterment of children while earning less than stellar pay. This has nothing to do with them and everything to do with the actual system. To say that the curriculum in our public schools is biased and built to condition is an understatement.

Elementary school is the foundation of the education system. From day one, the goal of the system is not to teach the individual to use their mind to understand the concept of learning, but to teach them how to follow authority through a standardized process. They're taught systems... not innovation. Subjects like science teach baseline principles with the sole intent of primitive thinking. Teacher talks about it... student listens and attempts to memorize... then takes a test... and moves on. Baseline principles create baseline thinkers. In elementary school, children are rarely taught objective viewpoints that challenge the standard.

This line of teaching generates a submissive student. And it's all by design. The goal was never to make you think and expand your mind... it's to create a society of submissive individuals who bow down to authority, never question anything and ultimately live their lives under the parameters of the system. Luckily, there are some that resist and break out of the proverbial chains of molding. But always remember, they don't need everybody... they only need the majority. Because the majority will always keep things the way that they are.

It doesn't stop with science. How about history? Why do you think public school curriculum chooses to indoctrinate the youth when it comes to the true history of America? Why aren't children taught the explicit genocide of slavery? Why don't schools teach the true character of our presidents? Our leaders?

A nation with something to hide is an insecure nation. The indoctrination that takes place in our school system is designed to miseducate.

Why don't they teach kids about credit? About the process of buying a home? Investments? Inflation? Equity? Why is economics an elective and usually only one semester? What about health?

At the time of the writing of this book, health class has been removed from a majority of schools or has been subjected to elective status. Health. The most vital part of our existence. And the worst part of it all... is the system has yet to take our mental health into account.

The fact that meditation is not taught in schools is by far one of the biggest travesties in the educational system. There is an overwhelming amount of statistical information to support how meditation and mindfulness impacts the overall well-being of an individual. Not to mention, statistics show that meditation introduced at childhood, shows exponential benefits to a child's brain and behavior.

From an article in *Forbes magazine* written by Alice G. Walton:

"A 2004 study found that children with ADHD who learned meditation with their parents twice weekly in a clinical setting, and kept practicing at home, had better concentration at school, among other benefits. Mindfulness-based cognitive therapy for children (MBCT-C) has also been shown to help improve attention and behavior problems, and reduce anxiety in kids who started out with high anxiety levels. A study in 2013 showed that in boys with ADHD, an eight-week training in mindfulness, significantly reduced hyperactive behaviors and improved concentration. Other studies have pointed to similar results, and more are currently underway to continue exploring the connection."

Meditation and other mindfulness exercises are still labeled pseudo-science. It doesn't fall under the umbrella of what society considers the standard.

In an article written by Samoon Ahmad M.D. in *Psychology Today*, he references a paper published in the American Journal of Psychiatry showing that mindfulness meditation significantly reduced anxiety and depression levels among the 22 participants in the study. Perhaps more importantly, 20 out of the 22 participants were still practicing the stress reduction techniques that they learned while undergoing the study at their three-month follow-up, while 21 of the 22 were still using mindfulness of breathing techniques in their daily lives.

This is all an effort to hold us back from reaching our highest and most optimal self. I didn't learn about meditation until I was thirty years old... and it happened by accident. I stumbled upon a guided meditation app on my phone, tried it on one of my lunch breaks, fell asleep for about 20 minutes and woke up feeling better than I had felt in years! That type of actualization should not have happened by chance.

The entire educational process is by design, from the authoritative teachers to the miseducation to suppression of the creative mind. It's all set up to mold you into a well-rounded conditioned citizen who abides by the concepts of society.

Take a look at the ideology of the "American Dream". It's merely a plan that promotes success on controlled terms. Go to school. Graduate. Then college... get hired by a major corporation. Get married. Have kids. Work for about 45–50 years in a job or profession that you don't really love, but have come to accept. Retire — and continue the cycle on to the next generation.

See, entrepreneurship is rarely promoted. Dreams are often met with what authority figures call "realistic expectations." Right around the time kids reach their mid-teens, they're introduced to systemic dream killers.

Maybe you have a passion for music. Maybe you always dreamed to be a writer. Society tells you and makes you believe that these are no-win situations and high-risk professions. Too often, kids are pushed toward trendy careers or what are considered stable jobs — overlooking passions, continuing to subdue and repress an individual's creativity.

We're all born with creativity. Yes, some are able to tap into it more than others, but creativity is within us all. Creativity spawns thought that exists outside of what would be perceived as the norm. Creativity is an aspect of our consciousness that connects directly with universal energy. It gives us the ability to see beyond what's visible in the physical realm. The powers that be know this... and by design, do everything in their immense power to vanquish our creative power at a young age.

The system is designed for you to decide what you want to do for the rest of your life by the age of eighteen, with your decision influenced to align with the rest of society. Think about that. Kids are cycled through a streamlined educational system that acts as a funnel to create workers in a corporate system. Fortunately, this couldn't be further from the truth. There are no time restraints on making life altering decisions. Time is a man-made construct that, once again, supports the systems put in place. This artificial pressure puts stress and anxiety on children... all by design.

Thou Shalt Not Be Conditioned

"Men are apt to be much more influenced by words than by the actual facts of the surrounding reality." - Ivan Pavlov

In the 1890s, Russian physiologist, Ivan Pavlov noticed that his dogs would begin salivating whenever they heard the footsteps of his assistant bringing them the food. The dogs associated any object or event that they associated with food with the same response. Footsteps. A clicking metronome. A bell. This became the foundation of what we know now as *Pavlovian conditioning*. An indirect programming of the mind that creates a stimulated response.

Now think about all the indirect programming you've received. No, I'm not talking about salivating at the mouth at the sound of a waiter's footsteps... this is deeper than that. Take a look at the media. The film industry. The music industry. Television. Magazines. Social media. They've taken Pavlovian conditioning to the next level.

The media has done an incredible job of creating the association of crime with people of color. That's not by accident nor is it factual. One of the most famous catch phrases in today's society is "black on black crime" as if it's truly an epidemic that stands on its own. In 2018, the Federal Bureau of Investigation reported that 81% of white victims were killed by white offenders, and 89% of Black victims were killed by Black offenders. How many times have you heard about "white on white crime"? You'd think an 8% difference wouldn't constitute such a varying depiction of culture. Yet, the majority of crime you hear about on the news is culturally biased. People kill the people they're around, simple and plain.

How does this associate with Pavlovian conditioning? Well...

Ivan Pavlov conducted his experiments by using the following terms. The unconditioned stimulus (food) which represented the event that produced a natural response (saliva) and the neutral stimulus (footsteps), in which by itself, did not produce a response. Once the neutral stimulus (footsteps) became associated with the unconditioned stimulus (food), it became a conditioned stimulus causing a conditioned response.

Now let's integrate my media analogy into the experiment.

The unconditioned stimulus would be crime. Crime in itself induces the natural response of fear. People of color represent the neutral stimulus, which by themselves, do not induce a fear response. The association of people of color and crime through the media creates a conditioned stimulus causing fear. There have been many studies that show people, black and brown included, are subconsciously more afraid of people of color than whites. This is by design.

Before the civil rights act in 1964, the portrayal of black and brown people by the majority of America was that of an inferior species. Society had free reign to depict people of color however they wanted on television, in books, magazines and in public. That inferior perception is another form of Pavlovian conditioning that was passed on for generations after the Atlantic Slave Trade.

The unconditioned stimulus was the social perception of blacks which induced the natural response of white superiority. Freedom was the neutral stimulus but when associated with the perception of blacks and their lack of freedom, also attributed to white superiority. Once people of color gained their freedoms, this specific conditioning didn't go away by any means, but it did lose some impact. The design didn't cease, it only shifted to attack the credibility of people of color in a more discreet way.

How do you attack the credibility of someone? By conditioning the way people perceive them. Associating black and brown people with crime attaches them to one of our most sensitive emotions; fear. Add in a justice system that was never created to protect society, but to placate those who have a specific perception of society, and you have another institution built on a foundation of bias.

The justice system in America is set-up to make you believe that individuals accused of a crime will be judged by a jury of his/her peers. Unfortunately, it is impossible for anyone — especially people whose character and credibility have been attacked for generations — to get a fair and just process. It's all by design. It's no coincidence that the majority of people who occupy the nation's prisons are people of color.

According to an article by John Gramlich of *pewresearch.org*, as of 2017, blacks represented 12% of the U.S. adult population but 33% of the sentenced prison population and Hispanics represented 16% of the adult population while accounting for 23% of inmates. Over half of the prison population are people of color while barely exceeding a quarter of the American populace.

Why? Let's dive deep into the design of this country.

When people reference the idea of "white privilege", it's not to offend or denigrate but to point out a mere fact. White people have had the advantage of a massive head start when it comes to generational ascendancy. That doesn't excuse anyone from the choices they make or the life they decide to live, but it does impact their environment and level of conditioning they receive.

Every system created within this country was designed to make the poor poorer, the rich richer and the middle class stagnant. From welfare, section 8 housing, and the federal housing administration to a financial system that preys on the lower to middle class, it's set up for the average person or family to be reliant upon them.

We're a product of our environment, right? If the majority of people of color are only a few generations removed from legislative inequality, it makes sense that they would represent the bulk of the lower social class in America. The aforementioned programs are conditioning devices to brainwash the lower social class into thinking they're put in place to help them.

Why do you think welfare programs have restrictions such as asset limits? Some states as low as $1000. It's the social paradox. Entice poor people to get on welfare while also discouraging them from saving money. So, if a person truly wants to get off of welfare and get ahead, they can't.

Most financial advisors would suggest an individual have at least 6 months reserves before purchasing a home. That would be impossible for someone on welfare. They'd basically have to make a choice between saving their money or receiving the government assistance. Is it starting to make sense now?

It doesn't stop there. The FHA mortgage program was created with this in mind. Don't have much money to put down on a home? No problem... you can get a home with as little as a 3.5% down payment!

Why is that a bad thing? Get a house with almost no money down! Once again... they've brainwashed people into thinking that mortgaging a home is true ownership. It used to be commonplace for a family to put at least 20% down on a home. This accomplished a number of things.

First, that meant when you bought a home, you would walk into equity. Real estate is one of, if not the best type of investment anyone can make. It also entices you to live in the home for a while, build up more equity and if you decide to sell one day, your investment would pay off tremendously. This goes back to generational ascendancy. It wasn't out of the question for families to live in their home for the entirety of the loan, then pass the home down from generation to generation while accumulating wealth.

Second, when you purchase a home with less than 20% down, you have to pay additional fees like mortgage insurance and pay a higher interest rate. Long story short, it's another example of a system built to make you think they're helping you when in actuality, they're helping themselves.

This all goes back to education. Buying a home is most likely the biggest purchase you'll ever make in your life, yet, it's barely mentioned in grade school. It should be a fundamental process for everyone. But if everyone knew the ins-and-outs of the financial system, they wouldn't be able to take advantage of us.

How many people know the purpose of a *truth-in-lending disclosure*? Better yet, how many bank employees or title companies go out of their way to explain it?

A *truth-in-lending disclosure* discloses the exact amount you're paying on your loan. Not the loan amount, but the exact amount of money that will come out of your pocket. For example, when you buy that car for $25,000 on a 72-month term at 6.99%, you're actually almost paying $31,000 for the vehicle.

It doesn't matter though, right? You needed a car... but this isn't about teaching you or anyone how to be financially responsible, it's about understanding how the systems and programs put in place are here to limit you, control you and keep you coming back for more.

Politics, religion, healthcare, banking, the educational system and justice system were all created with bias and ulterior motives. On the surface, they appear to be put in place to help you and build an infrastructure of a strong healthy society. When you dig deep, which we have, you start to realize that these systems were put in place to mold you and your mind into a conforming resource.

Who is "They"?

Financial institutions run this country... and it makes sense if you think about it because money, power and greed run this country. The banking system has integrated itself into every facet of society and once again, have made us think we need them.

If you have a job, most likely you're paid by direct-deposit. Want to buy a car, you'll need a loan. Want to start a business, you'll need an identification number for taxing, registration with your state, a business checking account, possibly a credit card or line of credit and possibly a business loan. House = mortgage. Banking is everywhere.

When you break down how a bank makes money, it's almost laughable how bad we're all being played. Banks take YOUR money that YOU deposit and either invest it or loan it out to other individuals to earn a sizable return, only to pay YOU a minimal amount of interest. Think about that. They've created a system that pretty much mandates us to loan them our money, basically interest-free, only to have them loan it back to us and make billions. Hmmm...

I used to work for a second-chance banking institution that preyed on the less fortunate. Second-chance banking means they would target people with bad credit who couldn't get approved at the big-name banks. They positioned their banking centers in Wal-Marts and grocery stores so they could take advantage of the walk-by traffic. We'd use marketing tools such as free food, snacks, candy and giveaway prizes to entice this specific demographic to bank with us.

Instead of educating these individuals, who obviously didn't know anything about banking, saving or investing, the mission was to open as many new accounts as possible. The bank also offered a feature that allowed customers to overdraft their account, sometimes up to $500, as long as they had direct deposit. I'm sure you can guess how that went. The kicker? Overdraft fees were $35 each and the fee wasn't just attached to the item specific to the overdraft, but every item that posted along side of it. The fees racked up and accounts were being charged-off left and right. Truth is, this is how a lot of banks work, just at different levels and using different concepts. We don't need banks... but we've been conditioned to believe we do.

So, who is at the forefront of all this conditioning?

Most people associate these systems with the government and while they have a major hand in continuing to implement the processes of the powers that be, they are not solely responsible.

Who are the powers that be? Who is "they"?

It's a question that I receive consistently and I always answer it the same way. You have to look at the world like a corporation. In fact, the United States is a corporation. At the top of a corporation, you have the board of directors who make all the decisions. These decisions are always for the betterment of the corporation, not the employees. We are the employees. Remember what Jordan Maxwell said, we're a human resource. From the moment we're born, we're in training. Once we're of age, we work, contribute to the system, pay taxes, reproduce, die and continue the cycle through our offspring.

This board of directors consists of the most powerful individuals and entities on the planet. They represent the elite. They have the majority of the wealth which gives them the majority of the power in this material realm.

I'll get push back from individuals who can't comprehend how this group of people could care less about us. It's really simple and expands upon my previous example. If you've ever worked for a corporation, you'll understand where I'm coming from. Like I said, the elites represent the board of directors. The rich and somewhat wealthy represent upper management, while the middle and lower classes represent middle management to the ground level. If the decision has to be made to shut down a specific division or lay off a portion of the staff, it's done with zero hesitation.

Do you honestly think the heads of these corporations truly care about Denise in the mailroom? Or Jamal in accounting? Or Hector in marketing? Or the 25,000 people on the chopping block because their quarterly numbers are 22% lower than initial projections? These are people's lives and livelihood, dangling in the hands of a group of money-hungry, greedy and selfish individuals. There is no empathy.

So how does that correlate with society?

Imagine you're at the top of the wealth food chain and a part of this elite group. Your world is completely different than the average person. You don't mingle with the average Joe and barely occupy the same habitat. Your problems consist of sustaining your wealth, power and traditions for generations to come. Just like the board of directors are only concerned about their company, the elites are only concerned about their well-being.

Resources becoming scarce? World over-populating? Power spreading too thin? No problem, we'll just create systems to ensure we stay in power by indoctrinating the majority of people into thinking we're helping them, when in actuality, we're taking away their ability to decipher the truth from deception.

Back to the corporation analogy... there is no empathy when it comes to impacting their livelihood. Is there a difference between laying 10,000 people off and depopulation? Of course! But the motive is the same.

Depopulation is happening as we speak. No, not in the Hollywood-esque way most expect it to be... but by misinformation, brainwashing and conditioning. By promoting toxic habits, false medical theories, and medicine. By suppressing information, dumbing down society and creating mindless zombies. By detaching us from the most important and powerful aspect of life; ourselves. All of it plays a part in the downfall of society.

I'm betting that all of this has you thinking now. Questioning everything you've been taught and everything you claim to know. I could write an entire book on the amount of conditioning we face on the daily. Religion, education, politics, sports, medicine, history, science and the justice system... it's all there in plain sight for the awakened.

It all starts with the acknowledgement. Recognizing that everything isn't as it seems.

There's a beauty in questioning everything. Using your own deductive reasoning and analysis to break down the world. Understanding the motives behind the systems that control society. Taking the time to do your own research. Dissecting theories and not taking everything at face value. That's what they want... a planet full of sheep who follow orders, remain submissive and question nothing.

Take some time to evaluate your life and understand all the ways you've been conditioned. Write it down. This is a major aspect of self-reflection and self-realization.

Why are we the way that we are?

See, conditioning has an effect on our personality flaws, insecurities, thoughts, mental health, physical health, happiness, purpose and overall outlook on life. Our subconscious is a powerful beast. The powers of this world have done a masterful job of manipulating our subconscious.

So, what now? You've acknowledged that you've been conditioned. What's next? The next step on your path towards a healthy life is to detox your mind and break free.

When I came to the realization of the truth about Christianity, my first response was anger. How could I spend so much of my life believing something that was not only fabricated, but attached to such a corrupt organization? No matter how many denominations of Christianity are birthed, they all either funnel up or have a link to Catholicism. The Catholic church was and still is a powerful entity.

The anger response is normal. I made it a point to argue, exploit and attack anyone who promoted or tried to justify Christianity. On my podcast, I'd have live debates with anyone who wanted to challenge my thoughts on religion. It was my life's mission to prove to everyone that Christianity and all religion were bullshit! This was my pride taking over. Low frequency action motivated by a massive amount of resentment towards the religious system. As I continued to grow on my journey, that resentment faded away.

Anger is a part of the process because it's an expression of built up emotion. Breaking your conditioning is work... lots and lots of work. Unfortunately, most people who acknowledge the conditioning never end up breaking the conditioning. But not you... you can see the bigger picture. Enlightenment. It's a beautiful thing.

So, it's okay to be angry about how you've been duped to think the world operates with your best interest at mind. Just understand, that it's a part of the progression and not foundational. The goal is to grow and we cannot grow motivated by low frequency action. This is imperative, especially when you're in the process of building a healthy life. You have to look at it like you're building from the ground up... and when we're building from scratch, we want to use the most optimal material.

Breaking conditioning is different for everybody because we all have unique minds and we've been conditioned in different ways. For me, breaking my conditioning started with my outlook on life. When I began questioning everything, I started noticing the effects my conditioning had on my life.

Before the birth of my youngest daughter Nadia, my wife and I decided to do some deep research on vaccines. We concluded that we did not want the government dictating the health of our daughter. If we were to get her vaccinated, it would be on our schedule. This consisted of understanding the diseases that were associated with the vaccines, the chemicals used and the overall risk versus reward. It took some time to find the right doctor for Nadia, but eventually we did.

Breaking conditioning isn't about anti-vaccination, it's about freethinking. It's about ensuring you're making the best choices for you and your family. Two months after Nadia was born, we made the conscious decision to become vegetarians. Through countless nights of research on food, nutrition and health, this was the best path for our family. I was raised on a majority meat diet and have had countless health issues such as irritable bowel syndrome, high-blood pressure, lactose intolerance, frequent headaches and eczema. By becoming vegetarians who rarely consumed dairy (only cheese) at the time, a lot of my ailments subsided. In addition, and in my opinion most importantly, we no longer support the slaughtering of innocent animals, deforestation and the countless other environmental/ethical effects associated with meat production.

A big part of my spirituality stems from becoming a vegetarian. I'll touch more on this later in the book, but for me personally, in order to connect with my higher-self, I always believed I would need to give up eating meat. Feed yourself life and you will receive life.

Once you break free and detox your life, things start to happen fast!

A month after becoming vegetarians, my wife and I were both laid off from our jobs. We worked for a major corporation making really good money at a job we both loved. This was life altering. We had just bought a new house and just had a baby. At the time, there weren't many other companies hiring for our positions and the severance package we received would only last a few months. Part of my conditioning was believing in the corporate system when it came to making a living. Guaranteed paycheck, benefits, and a false sense of security. I was brainwashed to follow the corporate path and suppress my true passions and gifts.

Since I was 12 years old, I've had an ability to write and create. It started with music and transitioned into film. Nothing made me happier than writing music, scripts or directing films. From the moment I got entangled into the corporate world, my passions for the arts took a secondary role. I never quit, but it never became the main thing. Being laid off was one of the most eye-opening experiences of my journey. I enjoyed my job. The culture was diverse, money was great and I loved the people! But I got comfortable.

The facade of corporate America was blinding me while my hunger to chase my dreams was slowly dissipating. Fortunately for me, the universe had different plans. Being laid off ended my attachment to the corporate system. While I ended up taking another corporate job with a smaller company, I would never allow myself to detach from my passions. The corporate job was necessary while my true passions and what I consider my purpose in life were my happiness. If I was never laid off, I'm not sure where I'd be today, but it doesn't matter because there are no coincidences.

When you're not where you're supposed to be, whether that be a job or relationship, the universe will intervene. After being laid off, my journey went into overdrive and the transformation was immense! It's like the job was my final association to the conditioned world. Everything was different, including my connection to the universe. The veil had been lifted. Ideas came in abundance. In a span of a few years, I created my own film company, released two short films, three documentaries, multiple commercials, two music videos, wrote a feature length script and created a podcast with over 100 episodes. This spawned into me finding my ultimate passion in life; natural health coaching.

When I used to make music, it was very ego-centric. I had this built up animosity that was showcased in almost every song I made. My sole purpose was to prove that I was better than the next artist. It lacked connectivity. Emotion. Resonance. All aspects of myself that I believe to be embedded into my character. So, when you listened to my music, you weren't getting me... you were getting my representative. I wasn't prepared to give you me.

My films have been a pure extension of my creative abilities. Being able to manipulate emotion through narrative. Art imitating life imitating art. The cycle of artistic expression.

But it took my podcast, Minds Like Mine's, to uncover my true calling. I'm a lightworker. My purpose is to lead, inspire and open minds. To promote freethought and share my experiences while I seek the truth. To connect with other freethinkers and be a resource for the collective consciousness of the world. Upon that journey, there is no more important aspect then your terrain. Both inner and outer. Mind, body and soul. It's all connected just like we're all connected.

That's the thing... everyone's journey is different. Breaking conditioning for you may be recognizing you're in the wrong job or relationship. It might be altering your mindset towards life. You might start questioning what you watch on television and alter what you consume. Maybe you'll stop attaching yourself to stuff that doesn't benefit you or the betterment of humanity. Or all of the above.

Breaking every bit of conditioning you've ever received is a tall task and could take decades... but the process is what truly counts. Ultimately, you'll find yourself. It takes looking at everything you've been taught and come to know with a new set of eyes. Unconditioned eyes. Studying the motives behind everything in society. Is it for the betterment of humanity? Or is there an alternative motive supporting the action?

Like I said at the beginning of this section, conditioning is by design. Remember, they don't want you to find yourself. Finding yourself means you'll be less reliant on their systems. These systems were put in place to diminish our sovereignty, create division while promoting conformity, and suppress our individuality.

They control our terrain by the generations of conditioning through various mediums. It's time to break free from the restraints of limited thinking, a powerless approach and most importantly, an unhealthy way of life.

Covid-1984

"Power is in tearing human minds to pieces and putting them together again in new shapes of your own choosing." - *George Orwell*

I debated with myself on whether or not I would speak about the COVID-19 pandemic in this book and I concluded that there's really no better example of conditioning then what has happened to society in the past few years. Now look, I understand there's been so much misinformation and so many confusing elements to COVID-19 that it's hard to really get a grasp on what's real and what's fake, but if you've read what I've written so far, you'll realize that it's all by design.

The ingredients to cook up this pandemic were put into place almost a century ago and it all starts with a belief system centered on health. I want you to put on your freethinking cap and let's dissect everything that's happened since the moment we heard about the coronavirus.

It took one week for the officials in China to already have a name and a full-blown theory of what was going on in Wuhan. If you think about it, it's actually incredible because the people that were coming in sick had pneumonia like symptoms and Wuhan is one of the most polluted places on the planet, yet medical officials already had a full-blown diagnosis within seven days. Now, let's backtrack a little bit. Agenda 201 was a major conference that brought together the highest of high when it comes to medical officials, corporate moguls like Bill Gates and other elites. In this conference, they conducted a simulation of a virus that spread throughout the world and put together plans on how they would operate if that happened.

Now, I'm sure there are people that will say that this is a mere coincidence but as you will learn throughout this book and throughout the time you hear me speak, there is no such thing as a coincidence. If you look at the individuals that were a part of Agenda 201, you will also see them as a major part of everything that transpired throughout the entire pandemic. Remember, conditioning is all about control and in order to control you have to be able to manipulate.

One of the key aspects of manipulation is to tap into the emotions of the individual. So, let's quickly go over everything that transpired throughout the pandemic. You had an abundance of fear mongering, a media narrative that was pushed onto society, and the implementation of new systems to not only control the narrative but also dictate the overall outcome. Let's break that down...

One of the true testaments of conditioning is to be able to hide things in plain sight. From the onset of COVID-19, the data provided to the public painted a completely different picture than what the media and the health officials were portraying based on the narrative that was pushed. COVID-19 was this massive deadly virus that could destroy our way of life while the numbers didn't match the story. We're talking about a virus that had a death rate of 1% amongst all people and a death rate of .2% of anybody less than 55 years old. The response from the political officials and health officials were not only to instill fear in the people but also control the people. This was done by mandates to make people stay home and also force companies into some really difficult employment decisions. This was done by mandates to force people to wear masks with absolutely zero science behind it. This was also done by one of the oldest conditioning tricks in the history of the world; division.

Once again, in order to condition people... in order to indoctrinate people... you have to play on their emotions. Religion mastered it, politics enhanced it, and COVID-19 was the pinnacle.

By instilling so much fear through so many channels, you had people acting on behalf of this plan while the truth was facing them in plain sight. They were so conditioned that they didn't even see it. And when you're talking about people being fearful and playing on the emotion of fear, it causes people to act irrational. The division was strong. Political division ran rampant.

Division is one of the oldest tricks in the book because it adds more low frequency energy to the collective consciousness of the world. See, the world itself has its own collective consciousness and operates at a certain frequency, so when you have division, hate, fear, struggle and stress, it brings down the entire frequency of the world. This is how wars formulate and negative forces take over. They use this lower frequency to manipulate indoctrinated and conditioned individuals.

Look, I'm not here to say that nobody was getting sick. What I am saying is that this particular pandemic was all created by design. This was all put in place. And if you're asking why would this be put in place, once again you have to look back at the origins of the systems that were put in place.

The medical system, big pharma and the insurance business is at the foundation of all of this. We've been conditioned and indoctrinated to believe certain theories and certain ways of life that are at the root of our fears when it comes to health and wellness. I'll dive much deeper into this in the next section, but understand that the way people reacted to this pandemic was just a continuation of indoctrination that we've received our entire lives.

This played into the division as well, because you have a majority of people who haven't realized they've been conditioned... haven't acknowledged their conditioning... haven't broken free from it... and aren't aware of what's hidden in plain sight. As a result, they view individuals who don't follow mandates—who are awakened and do understand truth—as a threat to their own safety and health.

So, what exactly was the goal with this entire COVID-19 pandemic? I advise all of you to read the book *"Covid-19: The Great Reset"* by Klaus Schwab, the founder and executive chairman of the World Economic Forum.

The first indication that this was all a set-up and a plan happened for me roughly around the end of March 2020. COVID-19 hadn't really had a presence worldwide until the end of March, yet the World Economic Forum had already created a complex detailed plan on the following:

-What was going to happen

-How it was going to affect our economy

-How it was going to divide people

-what to do in the event of misinformation

-5G and how it would complement the surveillance of society

-What to do in the event of a non-compliant society when it came to the vaccine

All of this before Covid-19 was truly a pandemic. The aforementioned book was published June 2020, merely three months after Covid-19 was even an issue.

Now, I'm not here to say that Klaus Schwab—along with his collection of individuals working for the World Economic Forum—isn't highly intelligent. But putting together such an extremely complex web of connections to almost everything happening in society (including things that haven't even truly occurred yet) feels a little far-fetched.

The conditioning went from instilling fear into the people to promoting an advantageous narrative... to building up the false representation of a magic vaccine to attacking the credibility of anybody who spoke out against the vaccine... to putting systems in place such as surveillance and fact checkers to issuing authoritative mandates. All of this was done in the name of public safety—when in reality, these were just additional methods of control. These are the new systems being put in place.

And the most creative aspect of it all? You—the people, the conditioned society—are okay with it. Now that is the ultimate conditioning.

My theory on why people are getting sick is the perfect segue to the next section of this book...

The coronavirus isn't contagious. In fact, it's not even a virus. The powers of this world are pumping some form of toxic element in the air and we are breathing it and consuming it to the point where our bodies are having a major detox event. I'm smart enough to realize that the highly funded private scientists of this world know how our body functions. This is why the sick are getting sicker and the healthy are barely affected. This is why it's more of a threat to the elderly and an absolute non-factor to children. This is also why the vaccinated are far more likely to get sick.

Toxins to combat toxins is a win-win situation for the minds behind Covid-19.

The worst part of all this is that I believe it was the precipice of something bigger. This was a test to see how society would react. This was also a test to see what percentage of the population they can control. Remember, they only need the majority. Roughly 65% of the world received at least one dose of the coronavirus vaccine. That's two-thirds of the entire planet. According to USA Facts.com, 81% of the people in the United States of America received at least one dose. 70% are fully vaccinated.

As long as they have the majority of people brainwashed, conditioned and operating with a group think mentality, they can sell us anything.

How do we overcome this madness? Take our power back and create a healthy life.

Part Two
Creating a Healthy Life

Terrain Theory vs. Germ Theory

"Health and disease are the same thing-vital action intended to preserve, maintain, and protect the body. There is no more reason for treating disease than there is for treating health."- Herbert Shelton N.D.

We, as people, take our body for granted. Unfortunately, most of us don't understand the power we withhold within ourselves. If I told you that our body was a self-healing, self-fulfilling, self-cleansing machine, you would probably think I was crazy. When I talk about a healthy terrain, I'm not only talking about the food you eat, I'm also talking about the company you keep, the environment you live in, and ultimately anything you allow into your personal energy field.

I have a basic philosophy, and it's very simple. I ask myself: *Is whatever I'm about to partake in for the betterment of me or the detriment of me?* Is it good for me, or is it toxic for me? And that goes for every aspect of life—your relationships, your career, and the food you eat.

Diet is one of the most sensitive topics in the world today. You have to ask yourself why? Why is it so sensitive? Why are people so sensitive when it comes to what they eat? Well, this is all by design. There have been systems put in place for a very long time that have conditioned us and so heavily indoctrinated us, that the idea of keeping a healthy terrain seems absurd. So, just like in our *Freeing Your Mind* section, you have to question everything. If you look at how the systems, in America particularly, are built they all coincide with each other. Let's take a look at the medical field.

Over a century ago, there was a debate between French chemist Louis Pasteur and French scientist Antoine Béchamp on the foundation of disease. Pasteur supported the germ theory while Béchamp advocated for the terrain theory. These were two completely different outlooks on health from two completely different perspectives. We've all been conditioned to believe in the germ theory, that billions of invisible pathogens are attacking our body at all times and it's up to our immune system to keep us safe. It also advocates for treatment of symptoms with medicine. Terrain theory puts the accountability on the individual. In the terrain theory, dis-ease comes from within, built up from an unclean terrain (your body) due to unhealthy eating habits, toxic exposure and in some cases disposition (genetics). Interestingly enough, nearing death, Louis Pasteur reversed course and concluded that the terrain theory is indeed the underlying cause of disease.

"It is the soil, not the seed."- Louis Pasteur

Germ theory is heavily supported by the idea of contagion, which means that one person can make another person sick. Now, you're probably saying, *"Oh yeah, of course—we see it all the time..."* But if you dive deep into the science behind the theory of contagion and the theory of germs, you quickly realize that none of this has actually been proven—hence why it's called a theory. The conditioning is so strong that the idea there's no such thing as a cold virus, or no such thing as a chickenpox virus, seems ridiculous. I mean, we have countless examples of contagion, right? That's kind of what we've been taught to know. But in essence, we can't spread sickness in the same vein that we cannot spread health.

As explained in *What Really Makes You Ill? – Why Everything You Thought You Knew About Disease Is Wrong*:

"During the 19th century, scientists who believed in the germ theory had been able to discover a variety of bacteria that appeared to be associated with a number of the diseases they were investigating. However, they were unable to find a bacterial or even fungal agent associated with some of those diseases. This led them to the belief that there had to be some other organism that was responsible for those other diseases. They believed that it must be an organism that was too small to be seen through the optical microscopes of the period."

You have to ask yourself this question. If you're looking to create a system similar to the medical system, similar to the pharmaceutical system and similar to the insurance system, which theory would you be more apt to adopt?

The terrain model teaches that the body is self-healing, and that what we call sickness is actually the body initiating a healing response to restore balance and health. The symptoms are actually the healing process. Let's return to the question of which theory the architects of our societal systems would be more likely to adopt. There's no money in the terrain theory. Why? Because if the terrain theory was adopted in society, big pharma, medicine and health insurance would not exist in its current capacity.

Health insurance would be a luxury. The medical system would be more of a resource than a necessity. Big pharma would no longer be big. That's not to say we would not need doctors or hospitals per se because there are instances where we do need medical help. But if people truly understood that they have the power to heal themselves—and that sickness is simply the result of an unhealthy terrain—there would be little need for insurance. It would become optional at best, reserved only for catastrophic events.

You wouldn't need those routine yearly or semi-annual doctor visits. You wouldn't rely on prescriptions to manage blood pressure or other chronic symptoms.

But the system that's been put in place—along with the deep indoctrination of society—has created a world where people believe they can eat whatever they want, live however they want, and simply fix the consequences with a pill... or balance it out with a workout and be fine. That's exactly why the terrain theory never stood a chance in America.

Germ theory is where the money is. The real kicker in the entire medical system lies in the education provided to our health professionals. Some of you might be thinking, "I trust my doctor—they went through years of schooling, and there's a reason they're in that profession." And I completely respect that perspective. But the unfortunate truth is that doctors and health professionals have been indoctrinated too.

In 1910, John D. Rockefeller, shortly after the Sherman Anti-Trust Act broke up his oil monopoly, teamed up with Andrew Carnegie to recruit a professor named Abraham Flexner to write the most influential medical document our world has ever seen. *The Flexner Report* created the standardization of medical education and is the foundation of the medical system in the modern world today. Prior to *The Flexner Report*, people had a conscious choice of healing with an estimated split between holistic and allopathic (using treatments to diagnose and treat disease) health care. Once the report was adopted as the gold standard of health, only the American Medical Association (founded by Rockefeller) could grant medical licenses. Practicing without a license could lead to imprisonment.

The ramifications of this report are endless. Everything from medical insurance and pharmaceuticals to the lack of credibility associated with alternative and holistic approaches to health have been impacted by Rockefeller's scheme.

In the succeeding decades, the U.S. has seen cancer, heart disease, diabetes and other terrain-based diseases rise to astronomical heights, creating continuous opportunities for the health care systems to capitalize monetarily.

"A pill for an ill" was the mantra associated with the Rockefeller health movement. It stands true today, as 75% of the advertising on tv, magazines and streaming are pharmaceutical based. In addition, the sale of pharmaceuticals accounted for over 550 billion dollars in 2022.

If the education that our health professionals are receiving is based on a *germ theory system* then it has nothing to do with intelligence and everything to do with knowledge within that specific system.

Another deep aspect of the indoctrination and conditioning is the fact that we've been trained to see doctors as authority figures. They're the experts, right? We've been programmed to submit to medical professionals without questioning their opinions. If you're reading this book, we have to eliminate that way of thinking. You are sovereign—you have every right to ask questions and question everything. This is your life, not the doctor's, not society's, not anybody else's but yours.

Did you know it wasn't until 1985 that the *National Academy of Sciences* recommended nutritional education in medical school? The key word is "recommended," implying it's optional for each school. What's even more mind-boggling is that only 25 hours are suggested.

A survey of U.S. Medical Schools in 2010 found that only 27% of programs met that recommendation.

Umm, what?

Another survey of medical schools published in the *Journal of Human Nutrition and Dietetics*, found that most students in the U.S. and U.K. receive an average of 11 hours of nutrition training throughout an entire medical program. Part of this training is typically student-run, and it may include culinary classes.

The Flexner Report helped create a society where health is a byproduct of medical care as opposed to nutrition and diet. Effects include the creation of the standard American diet which has been adopted by both the healthcare system and the educational system as the gold standard of nutrition.

Who remembers the food pyramid? You know, the upside-down funnel that advocates for 6-11 servings of breads, cereal, rice and pasta while only 2-4 servings of fruit. These are the people we're trusting with our livelihood.

When you start to look at health from a systemic point of view, you'll quickly realize how it all ties together and how it's not for the betterment of your livelihood.

What to E.A.T.?

"If the human body is electrical, then the nourishment should also be electrical." - Dr. Sebi

Let's dive deeper into the terrain model. If the basis of the terrain model is the cleanliness of your inner-terrain/body, then the foundation of the model is your diet. It all starts with the same basic principle and philosophy: Is what I am consuming for the betterment of me or the detriment of me?

When it comes to diet, there is no middle ground. As humans, we all have something called vital energy or vitality and that energy is what keeps our body functioning. The fuel for that energy is carbohydrates, and the optimal fuel is natural carbohydrates. The natural diet is the only diet that is truly beneficial for you and consists of raw fruits, veggie fruits, leafy tender greens, nuts and seeds. The body is able to absorb the nutrients and digest these foods without expelling too much energy, lifting the burden from the body during the metabolic process and allowing for the absorbed energy to be utilized for the body's greater good. They cover all nutritional needs and a healthy combination of these foods will yield a clean well-balanced terrain.

Every food outside of the natural diet would be considered foreign to the body and otherwise toxic. Now, there are different levels of toxicity, but it's important to know that foreign foods put a higher level of burden on the body and do not offer enough energy to compensate for the burden. This is what I call energy efficiency, which is the first pillar in my E.A.T. philosophy. It's your body's profit & loss system.

E.A.T. stands for energy efficiency, avoid acid-forming foods and toxicity. They all work in tandem with each other to create a healthier you.

When it comes to energy efficiency, here's a breakdown of foods from most efficient to least efficient:

ENERGY EFFICIENT (a positive net energy exchange)
Fruits
Leafy greens, veggie fruits, nuts & seeds

NOT ENERGY EFFICIENT (a negative net energy exchange)
Cooked veggies, plant starch
Starches
Dairy
Meat/Fish
Processed foods

Why is energy efficiency so important? To keep it simple, like I mentioned earlier, we are a self-healing and self-cleaning organism. Our body, through our autonomic nervous system, utilizes available nerve energy to clean, heal and repair our inner-terrain. The more energy our body has at its disposal, the more healing can occur. The body's number one goal is to survive and achieve balance or homeostasis. Through conditioning, indoctrination and programming, our inner-terrain's been abused for generations with poor eating habits and environmental toxicity.

Each one of us have different genetic weaknesses. Despite what we've been told by the medical community, these weaknesses can be healed. The disease you've been diagnosed with can be cured.

It starts with your diet and energy efficiency. This is why water fasting is so powerful. Consuming water doesn't trigger the digestive process, allowing the body a full gamut of energy for healing. Digestion is the most taxing process on the body and requires the most energy, which is why it's so vital to be energy efficient in your dietary choices.

We are frugivores by nature. Meat is foreign and toxic. Fish is foreign and toxic. Processed foods are foreign and toxic. Dairy is foreign and toxic. Any cooked food is foreign and toxic.

What? Even cooked vegetables? Yes.

When we cook our food, not only are we adding additional toxic elements to the food through the cooking process, we're actually reducing the amount of nutrients as well. Nutrient degradation starts at 120 degrees. Now, think about the level of temperatures you use to cook your food. That goes for any and all cooked, grilled, baked, roasted and even pasteurized foods. As soon as heat is added to the equation, the chemistry of the food changes.

From Dr. Douglas N. Graham's *The 80/10/10 Diet*:

"Heating fuses foods into molecules our digestive system cannot easily process. Cooking denatures the proteins in foods, fusing the amino acids together with enzyme-resistant bonds that prevent them from being fully broken down, rendering the proteins substantially useless and, in fact, toxic to us. The digestion of cooked complex carbohydrates is typically impaired by the fatty and sugary foods with which they are consumed, leading to fermentation. The byproducts of fermentation are gas, alcohol, and acetic acid. Alcohol is a protoplasmic poison that kills every cell it contacts, and acetic acid is a known poison. Once fats have been cooked, they quickly go rancid, at which point they become carcinogenic."

I know a lot of people debate on our natural diet, but our physiology tells us what we're supposed to eat and what we've been designed to eat.

"After the discovery of vitamins, humans should have had the common sense to recognize how cooking disintegrates those vitamins. They should have put an end to that waste once and for all and safeguarded natural foodstuffs from degeneration. Is it not foolishness to burn and destroy those essential constituents by one's own hands, to become ill, to stand on the brink of the grave, and then make hopeless attempts to save oneself by deceptive means?"
— from the book *Nature's First Law: The Raw Food Diet* written by Stephen Arlin, Fouad Dini and David Wolfe

People ask me all the time how civilization survived if they weren't able to eat meat. We need to look at this from a consciousness perspective. Our earliest recorded ancestors came from Africa, and Africa, with its tropical climate, was able to provide humans with an assortment of natural vegetation. Some of the civilization eventually migrated north into Europe to colder climates where the assortment of fruits were not available. For survival, civilizations began eating meat.

The key word is survival. These civilizations were in survival consciousness. What separates us from the animals are levels of consciousness. Animals are in a survival consciousness, where their only intent is to eat, survive and procreate. We, as humans, have evolved to a higher level of consciousness and therefore have the choice of what we ingest into our bodies. That's not even mentioning the spiritual aspect, in which I'll touch on in a bit.

So, in summary, the adaptation of eating meat came from the migration of civilizations to colder climates and was brought upon for survival. If you look at how our bodies are physiologically built, from our teeth to our hands and to our intestines, you will see a major contrast compared to carnivores, omnivores and herbivores. Take this example, if you were to put me in a room with a cow and no weapons, would I be able to kill and eat that cow? The answer is obviously no.

We as humans were designed to eat the foods provided by the earth that correspond with our physiology. We have hands to grab fruits from trees. Since our jaws are not as strong as say a horse or a cow, we have to have a slight puncturing canine tooth to bite into certain fruits. Our intestines are not built to process meat. Meat resides in our system and can take anywhere from 8 to 24 hours to digest. This goes back to energy efficiency. That's a heavy burden on the body with little to no energetic return. This is why you feel tired, experience crashes or food comas after consuming meat. The moment an animal is slaughtered, the vital energy within that animal begins to deteriorate. So, in essence, there's more energy in a raw, freshly killed animal than a store-bought cooked piece of meat.

According to Dr. Robert Morse in *The Detox Miracle Sourcebook*, "The electromagnetic energy of cooked foods is dramatically lower than that of raw foods due to the change in molecular structure from the heat application... With heat, unsaturated fats become saturated and many dangerous and carcinogenic compounds are created. Heat also destroys the enzymes in food."

Raw fruits and vegetables are the most electric foods on the planet and we are electrical beings. Electromagnetic energy is measured by angstroms. Fresh raw fruits and vegetables have anywhere between 8,000-10,000 angstroms of energy. Cooked veggies have half of that. Dairy has about one-fifth while cooked meat has zero. A healthy terrain is an energy efficient terrain. *How much energy is the food giving me versus how much energy is being exerted in the digestion process?*

Dr. Morse also talks about two sides of chemistry; hot and cold. Acid and alkaline which is in line with my E.A.T. philosophy. In order to maintain a healthy terrain, you want to consume more alkaline-forming foods than acid. The more acid-forming foods you eat, like cooked meals, meats, refined sugars, starches, sodas, alcohol etc., the more likely you'll be prone to disease in the body. Acids are corrosive and destructive. Alkalinity is regenerative. The natural diet is alkaline dominant.

There are so many additional aspects to the understanding of the body and why the natural diet is the gold-standard of health, but my focus of this book is on helping you open your mind. Remember, in order to detox yourself, you have to fully comprehend how you've been intoxicated.

Getting healthy and transitioning to a healthy lifestyle is a process. That's why I always tell my clients that I will meet them where they're at. Do I expect everyone who reads this book to become a frugivore?

Not in the slightest... at the moment of writing this book, about 90% of my diet is natural. I'm not perfect by any means. But, I have experienced dramatic changes to my life by implementing my philosophies and concepts. It's about learning how your body works and hopefully this book can influence you to make some changes to your habits. Introduce more raw whole foods into your diet and watch your body change!

It starts with simple transitions. If you're currently eating 90% cooked food compared to 10% raw, focus on getting to 80-20. Take incremental steps towards a healthier you. Intention is powerful, so the moment you make your diet a priority, your body will start to adapt.

One of my biggest concerns with transitioning to a majority raw plant-based diet was the fear of missing out on the foods I had grown to love. I must say, this was one of the biggest a-ha moments for me on my journey to a healthier life. Your palette changes. Once you introduce living vibrant fresh whole foods to your diet, your body responds quickly. You'll be able to tell the difference.

When I'm coaching, I always tell my clients to record how they feel during and immediately after they consume foods from the natural diet compared to when they eat cooked food. It's an amazing contrast. It's like your body is awakened after decades of deep sleep. This is the electricity Dr. Morse talks about. You'll get addicted to this feeling and more importantly, as you continue, you'll get addicted to the healing.

Will you still crave cooked foods? Meats? Starches? Sugar? Yes. But the longer you continue implementing natural eating habits, the smaller the cravings.

Be sure to give yourself grace. Changing your eating habits after decades of a poor diet can be an extremely rough transition for some. It starts with the mind. Meditation can do wonders when it comes to dealing with cravings and relapses. Focus on the process and know that the body is always trying to heal itself. As you get further down the path of a healthy diet, your body will start speaking to you. If you've been consuming mostly cooked food your entire life, your body has built a tolerance to the toxicity. Once you start adjusting those cooked-to-raw ratios, that tolerance will diminish and your overall awareness of how your body feels after each meal will increase. It's no different than consuming alcohol. After years and years of drinking, you build up a tolerance to the poison and are able to consume more and more with little to no effect. Once you stop drinking for a while, your tolerance diminishes and now you're puking your guts out.

Is this crazy guy comparing eating cooked food to alcohol? Yes. Look, it's all chemistry and both are toxic to the body. Both are for the detriment of you. Different levels? Yes, but eating majority cooked meat, dairy, starches, fish and processed food will ultimately lead to some or many forms of dis-ease within the body.

A Toxic Body is an Angry Body

"What we suppress today is your nightmare tomorrow."
- Dr. Robert Morse

It took me three decades to realize I was on the wrong path. I always had a fascination with the natural diet. Even as a child growing up, I was drawn to trying to understand the belief system behind veganism and vegetarianism. Now, through a lot of generational conditioning, as well as societal conditioning, my diet was pretty bad. Heavy meats, lots of potatoes and grains, a bowl of cereal before bed and way too much dairy. I didn't understand the ramifications of the food I ate besides gaining weight.

Society teaches us that everything is about weight. Nothing else. Eat whatever you want, just don't let your weight get out of control. Once I started my healing journey, I always had this feeling that the best path towards enlightenment was to only consume life and remove death from my diet. Through my studies of Hinduism, Buddhism and Syncretism, I made the personal decision that my journey would continue by removing the consumption of living creatures from my lifestyle. It wasn't easy, but with the support of my wife, it was feasible.

There's a spiritual aspect to your diet as well. The act of slaughtering another conscious earth roaming creature has energetic consequences in my opinion. I feel that most meat-eaters operate on an *out of sight, out of mind* philosophy. Meaning, since they are *not doing the slaughtering*, they are without guilt or blame... or *since the animals are going to be killed anyway*, what's the difference if they decide to eat them? Some people feel that animals were put on this earth for our consumption and for our resources. This philosophy is directly linked to religious indoctrination.

Once you realize that everything conscious is connected, you quickly realize why the killing of animals for consumption is selfish and irresponsible. Not to mention, the effects it has on your terrain.

We've been conditioned to think that we need animal protein to not only survive, but thrive. This way of thinking has caused most people to disconnect from their natural instincts and inner-self. Now, by no means am I saying that you cannot be spiritual or thrive spiritually if you consume meat. I am merely giving you my thought process and philosophy on what has been a major foundation of my own spiritual growth. The motive behind this book is to make you think, look within yourself and question everything. Remember, the decision is always yours and my experiences illustrated in this book are here to provide guidance.

Whenever you're deciding on what you should eat, ask yourself these three questions: How much energy is the food giving me? How much energy is the food taking from me? And lastly, is the food acid-forming or alkaline-forming? If you start focusing your diet on those three questions, you'll get yourself on the path towards a healthier terrain.

An unhealthy terrain is a breeding ground for sickness. Through generations of misinformation and indoctrination, our ancestors have passed down bad eating habits that have ultimately contributed to society's demise. If you look at the leading causes of death in America, the top three are terrain-based diseases; heart disease, cancer and medicine. Now, medicine won't show up on a CDC list for leading causes of death, but medicine is a huge contributing factor to what causes us, our bodies, to break down.

According to analysis published in the *BMJ* *(formerly the British Medical Journal)*, medical errors claim the lives of 251,000 Americans each year. This puts it higher on the list than accidents, strokes, respiratory disease, Alzheimer's and more. The only conditions that cause more deaths are heart disease and cancer.

Medicine is toxic for your body. You need to look at medicine in the same vein that you look at food. It does not pass any of my basic philosophies. Medicine is toxic. Medicine does not provide any energy to you. Medicine taxes the body. Medicine is on the acid-forming side of chemistry. Lastly and most importantly, medicine suppresses the natural healing function of the body. It's merely a Band-Aid to help suppress a symptom or symptoms.

If the symptoms are evidence of the body healing itself, then the medicine is doing more harm than good. By suppressing the symptoms and stopping the body from healing itself, the eliminative toxins are never removed and end up accumulating within the terrain.

The medical system takes a reactive approach to health, while the terrain model focuses on a proactive approach. Doctors treat symptoms. I'm helping you understand the reasoning behind the symptoms and the eventual cure.

The truth is, there is only one cause of dis-ease within the body and that is acidosis. The build-up of acids within the body cause a chemical imbalance which ultimately manifests into a plethora of different systemic reactions. These reactions are the either the body's response in an effort to clean, remove and heal the body on its path back to homeostasis/balance or the effect of systemic breakdown.

According to Harvey Diamond in his book *Fit for Life*, disease progresses through seven distinct stages:

1.. **Enervation** - occurs when the body doesn't generate enough energy for its necessary functions or when the demands placed on it exceed its energy supply. Since sleep restores our energy, the first signs of enervation include feeling tired, sluggish, needing naps during the day, or requiring more sleep at night.

2.. **Toxemia** - the body becomes overwhelmed with toxins due to the continued abuses from the first stage. The organs responsible for detoxification—like the intestines, liver, kidneys, skin, blood circulation, and lymphatic system—become clogged and less efficient. As more energy is diverted to digest harmful substances and stimulants (such as coffee, alcohol, sugar, and tobacco), the body's cellular energy declines. This results in intoxication, sluggishness, weakness, and increased susceptibility to disease. A universal symptom of toxemia is fever, which is the body's attempt to eliminate excess toxins. It's important to allow the fever to run its course naturally, supporting the body by staying hydrated and resting.

3.. **Irritation** - the body activates its defense mechanisms to expel stored toxins, leading to various warning symptoms:
- Itchy skin

- Persistent tickling in the nose
- Feelings of irritability or restlessness
- Nervousness, depression, or anxiety
- Difficulty sleeping
- Unexplained weight gain
- Coated tongue, bad breath, increased body odor
- Sallow complexion or dark circles under the eyes
- Unusual menstrual issues

4.. **Inflammation** - the body's intensified effort to cleanse and heal itself, often accompanied by pain. This process indicates that toxins have been concentrated in a specific area for elimination, causing inflammation due to constant irritation. Common inflammatory conditions include various "itises" like tonsillitis (inflammation of the tonsils) and arthritis (inflammation of the joints). Skin conditions like eczema and psoriasis are examples of the body pushing toxins out through the skin.

5.. **Ulceration** - the body has been under prolonged assault, massive amounts of cells and tissues are destroyed, leading to ulceration. This condition is often painful due to exposed nerves and can result in lesions or ulcers both internally and externally. While the body may use ulcers to eliminate toxins, healing can occur if the toxic load is sufficiently reduced.

6.. **Induration** - involves the hardening of tissue or the formation of scar tissue where it has been lost. This hardening serves to encapsulate toxic materials, effectively quarantining them to prevent further harm. These sacs or tumors are the body's way of isolating toxins. If harmful practices continue, cells may begin to behave abnormally, leading to more serious conditions like cancer.

7..   **Cancer** - In the final stage, cells undergo genetic changes due to repeated damage from toxins and free radicals. This leads to uncontrolled cell proliferation and mutations, resulting in cancerous growths. At this point, cells no longer function properly or contribute to the body's well-being.

In summary, these seven progressive stages represent the body's attempts to restore balance and eliminate toxins. What we often label as "disease" is, in essence, the body's natural healing process working to correct internal imbalances. Recognizing and addressing the root causes at each stage can support the body's efforts to heal and maintain health.

What causes the body to progress from acute sickness to chronic dis-ease? Let's keep it simple.

What does health look like?

Health is balance within the body — every aspect working in harmony as it was intended. No burden. No struggle. No dis-ease.

If we had a perfect human being, this is how they would function: Our perfect human would live in harmony, eat food provided from a non-toxic earth to fulfill his/her hunger and provide energy to perform his/her normal functions. The food would be quickly broken down, nutrients transitioned thru the blood to the cells and the digestive waste quickly removed shortly after. The cells would consume the nutrients, generate energy and then their wastes would be quickly removed thru the lymphatic system. This cycle would continue and our perfect human would experience optimal life with no sicknesses, dis-ease, ailments or internal weaknesses.

Unfortunately, we don't live in a perfect world and neither did our ancestors.

Our conception is basically a cellular snapshot of our parents. That, along with our mother's internal terrain and habits during the gestation period determine our genetic disposition at birth. Some of us are born with a weak liver. Some of us are born with a weak pancreas. Some of us are born with a multitude of genetic weaknesses.

Long story short, we start life with a deficit.

This can be reversed, but our lack of understanding is the biggest issue facing mankind. We have to be extra conscientious of the toxins that surround us and accompany our food. We have to eat the foods designed for our body, so we can take advantage of our body's healing abilities. We have to consume hydrating alkaline-dominant foods so our lymphatic system can flow smoothly and remove toxins from the body. A healthy free-flowing lymphatic system is imperative to a healthy terrain.

"The physical body is a city unto itself... The lymphatic system picks up the trash from each house in the city (each cell); trash will vary, of course, depending upon the "lifestyle" within each house/cell and keeps your body clean... many foods that people routinely eat clog and over-burden the lymphatic system. Colds, flu, allergies, sinus congestion, bronchitis, lung issues-including pneumonia and asthma (with adrenal weakness)- along with mumps, tumors, boils, lymphomas, skin rashes, dandruff, etc... are nothing more than an over-burdened, congested lymph system." - Dr. Robert Morse from his book *The Detox Miracle Sourcebook*.

When we eat a majority cooked food diet that consists of meats, starches, processed foods and dairy, we prohibit our bodies from functioning the way they were intended to. The food is not quickly broken down, instead it sits in our digestive system requiring multiple processes from different organs just to salvage any semblance of nutrition for our cells. This depletes our vital energy, causing an energetic imbalance and fatigue. Digestive waste accumulates throughout our GI tract and constipation occurs due to the lack of hydration from the dehydrating foods. Remember, in a perfect world, we would be experiencing a bowel movement shortly after every meal. Our cells receive inadequate nutrition which in turn produce inadequate energy. Cellular waste, debris and acid ash accrue in the lymphatic system causing stagnation and build up in the interstitial spaces of the body. As this vicious cycle continues, the body breaks down, lacking the nerve energy to heal itself resulting in the aforementioned stages of dis-ease within the body.

Medical Malpractice

"The doctor of the future will give no medicine, but will interest his patient in the care of the human frame, in diet and in the cause and prevention of disease." - Thomas Edison

One of the biggest foundation pieces of the germ theory are viruses. Viruses have become a normal aspect of life for most of us. But when you take a look at the history of science and medical research concerning viruses you will see some gaping holes, shaky science and weathered theories.

Centuries ago, when someone got sick, the general consensus was that something spiritual was at play—a demon or dark energy had taken over the body. It sounds crazy, but in essence, it's very similar to the virus theory. Since most of us have taken everything we've been told by the medical industry at face value, it's hard to imagine that viruses and bacteria don't actually make us sick. This, in turn, makes it difficult to believe that our bodies are self-healing. Let me put it this way: without any knowledge of medical or scientific research, how would you try to prove that a virus could not only spread from person to person but also make that person sick?

Breaking everything down to its most basic element, you would first identify the virus in the sick individual, extract it, implant it into another individual, and see if it makes that person sick. Now, these experiments don't take place with humans due to medical ethics—it's considered unethical to experiment on human subjects. But even if you examine every virus ever claimed and how their conclusions were reached, you'll see that these basic principles were never followed.

Koch's postulates are essentially a set of guidelines that help us identify whether a specific microorganism is the cause of a particular disease. Think of them as the detective's rulebook for tracking down the culprit behind an illness. Here's a straightforward breakdown:

Consistent Presence: The microorganism must be found in every case of the disease but not in healthy individuals. This means if someone is sick, this germ is always there; if they're healthy, it's not. It's like noticing that every time a cookie goes missing, the same kid has crumbs on his shirt.

Isolation and Growth: We should be able to isolate this germ from the sick person and grow it in a pure culture. In other words, we take the suspect germ and see if we can nurture it independently to confirm its identity—much like taking fingerprints to match them later.

Reproduction of Disease: When we introduce this cultured germ into a healthy individual, it should cause the same disease. This step is crucial because it shows that the germ isn't just present during illness but actually causes it—similar to testing if a key opens a specific lock.

Re-isolation: Finally, we must be able to re-isolate the same microorganism from the newly infected host. This confirms that the germ we introduced is the same one causing the disease, closing the case with solid evidence.

The medical industry can't even support step one. Their justification? Well, people can be asymptomatic. Just another attempt to cover their bases.

Viruses and bacteria are merely solvents. They are elements that are a vital part of the healing and detoxing process of the body. Just because they are present when a sickness, disease or in our case, healing event, does not mean they are the cause of the sickness. This is an assumption and theory based on faulty science. If you look at most of the viruses and sicknesses in general, you will see that they share most of the same symptoms. Also, if you look at the testing and how the diagnosis is made by a doctor, you'll uncover even more holes.

There's no better example of this shaky science than HIV and its eventual cause of AIDS. According to medical professionals, the HIV virus can lay dormant in your body for years.

According to the *CDC fact sheet for AIDS/HIV*, "HIV Infection is often diagnosed through rapid diagnostic tests, which detect the presence or absence of HIV Antibodies."

This is a complete contradiction to both vaccines and normal medical practice. Antibodies, supposedly, are created by the body in response to a pathogen. Sort of like a blueprint of the pathogen, creating a defense system against the pathogen if it ever were to enter the body again. Vaccines, supposedly, replicate a pathogen to induce the antibody response. If an individual takes an HIV test and comes back HIV positive, then according to modern medicine, HIV would not be able to survive in the body.

This is where the medical system attempts to cover their bases once again. Supposedly, there are two completely different ways antibodies are interpreted. One is for protection, supporting my aforementioned summary of antibodies. The other is to indicate infection, which supports the HIV correlation to AIDS.

If you visit the home page of the Virus Myth website, you'll see a statement by Dr. Mullis that states, "If there is evidence that HIV causes AIDS, there should be scientific documents which either singly or collectively demonstrate that fact, at least with a high probability. There is no such document."

The entire AIDS epidemic is just another byproduct of how much power the medical system has on society. AIDS isn't the first disease to indoctrinate the minds of individuals, but before Covid-19, it was the most impactful. People don't remember that AIDS was originally called the gay disease. Gays were checking themselves into hospitals at rapid rates in the late 70s and early 80s and doctors had no answer nor diagnosis for what was going on. Symptoms included sores in the genital area, infection of the lymph glands, pneumonia... coincidentally, the same symptoms mirror those of syphilis.

Vaccines have always been a touchy subject. Based on the healthcare system put in place, the idea of a vaccine sounds amazing. A breakthrough that could ultimately bring health and wellness to humanity. Let's be honest, nobody enjoys being sick. So, if modern day science can create a magic elixir to stop us from being sick or suffering from disease, we'd be all in. Here's the issue...

Regardless of where you come out on vaccines, relying on vaccines for health is backwards thinking. Even If you believe that germs are constantly attacking us and you subscribe to the germ theory, vaccines act as a crutch to the overall healthcare system. Vaccines, as well as the majority of modern-day medicine, only promote reliance instead of being proactive towards your health. Now, we can continue to have a lengthy discussion on whether or not contagion exists, but that's not what this book is about. My goal is to help you understand the true meaning of a healthy terrain.

Whatever way you want to slice it, vaccines are toxic. They are made of toxic materials. So, when we're looking at the basic philosophy of consuming non-toxic food that gives you high levels of energy while minimally taxing the body, vaccines do not pass the test. The body is self-healing. Disease cannot exist in a healthy, thriving terrain. Adding additional toxic chemicals to your body makes zero sense when the goal is to rid the body of toxins. That's why vaccines have been so heavily debated to this day.

The rise in cognitive diseases and disorder, including autism, have been linked to vaccines in numerous scientific reports. Unfortunately, we don't always see these reports due to the indoctrination of society. Remember, there's a lot of money in medicine and vaccines are the golden goose.

Some may say that there's no direct link between vaccines and autism or other cognitive disabilities, but like I said earlier, due to the inability to track the long-term effects of a vaccine, we have to look at trends. The trends and data show a severe increase in cognitive issues at the same time as the increase of suggested vaccinations.

At the end of the day, whether or not you choose to get yourself or your family vaccinated is a private issue, not a public issue.

One of the biggest misconceptions, especially during Covid-19, is that a vaccine can stop contagion. This is where indoctrination and groupthink have infiltrated society's intelligence. Government agencies across the world made it a point to spread misinformation regarding the Covid-19 vaccine and made it a public issue. However, how you decide to treat your body or your family's body is 100% your choice and that's how it should be.

The Conscious Choice

"Change is inevitable but transformation is by conscious choice." - Heather Ash Amara

Another aspect of a healthy terrain is your living environment. This is often overlooked and sometimes referred to as pseudoscience, but the correlation between electromagnetic frequencies, electricity and your health is unquestioned. We are electrical beings.

I implore each and every one of you to read the book *The Invisible Rainbow: A History of Electricity and Life* by Arthur Firstenberg, to get a true grasp of how electricity impacts our health. As we progress technologically, we also digress both spiritually and biologically. Everything—from your cell phone, Wi-Fi, and computer screens to the appliances in your house, smart meters, 5G, Alexa, Siri, and LED lights—all combine to have detrimental effects on your health.

Many individuals have reported experiencing a range of minor symptoms that can be linked to exposure to electromagnetic frequencies. These can include persistent headaches, unexplained fatigue, sleep disturbances, difficulty concentrating, mood swings, and even feelings of anxiety.

Additionally, prolonged exposure to electromagnetic frequencies has been linked to more serious health conditions. Some research suggests associations between EMF exposure and diseases such as certain types of cancer, including leukemia and brain tumors. Neurological disorders like Alzheimer's and Parkinson's disease have also been explored in relation to EMF toxicity. Cardiovascular issues and fertility problems are other concerns that have emerged in scientific studies. It's crucial to recognize that our constant immersion in these invisible fields may be silently undermining our health. By becoming aware of these potential risks, we can take proactive steps to minimize our exposure and protect our well-being.

From the terrain perspective, your body is up to 75% water. EMFs emitting electromagnetic radiation are consistently and slowly cooking you internally. That may sound silly, but in essence, that's what's happening.

Per the *World Health Organization (WHO)*, "The main effect of radiofrequency electromagnetic fields is heating of body tissues."

Hydration is essential to health, which coincides with the alkaline-dominant water rich natural diet. Heat removes water. Consistent exposure to all of the aforementioned electricity will play a role in your overall health and terrain.

So how do you escape a world that's become reliant on electricity? The truth is, it is very difficult. But, there are things you can put in place to protect as much of your terrain as possible. When we built my current home, we had the builder install ethernet outlets in every single room with the intent of having a Wi-Fi free house. Now, for some this may be a huge inconvenience, but you have to weigh these things out. Is the convenience of having a Wi-Fi infiltrated home more important than your health? There have been many studies around cell phones, Wi-Fi and the newly introduced 5G that support significant health concerns. Once again, these are choices that you have to make.

It took me a while to realize that I was being severely affected by electromagnetic frequencies.

Due to my rigorous schedule of content creation, I am around computers and my phone the majority of the day. I began noticing massive headaches the longer I was subjected to my computer and phone. After doing a lot of research, I decided to shut off my Wi-Fi and see how I felt. In addition, I started turning my phone to airplane mode when I slept. The results were incredible.

First, my sleeping experience improved dramatically. Prior to switching my phone into airplane mode, I would wake up multiple times in the middle of the night, sometimes wake up with headaches and often wake up in the morning depleted of energy. Once I started sleeping without the electromagnetic frequencies constantly hovering around me, I was able to sleep through the night and woke up feeling 100% better. As for work, the headaches subsided tremendously with the occasional eyestrain headache from too much screen time, but overall, I have felt much better. To me, the trade-off is a no-brainer.

Control what you can control. We are living in a time where everything is becoming digitized. There's a major push for electric vehicles to be the standard. Most new vehicles today run off of computer software and are Wi-Fi ready. If we continue to stay subservient and not speak up, we're going to find ourselves swimming in an electromagnetic frequency stew. That's not to say that fuel-based cars don't cause environmental issues. The pollution and quality of air that we breathe is not optimal by any means. But, two wrongs don't make a right.

I'd be remiss to mention the importance of exercise and movement. When it comes to our physical health, exercise is a non-negotiable. In a *keeping it simple* fashion, when it comes to the body, you either use it or lose it. Most people have been conditioned to think that outside sources like protein powder and supplements can help them achieve physical health, but in actuality they cause more harm than good. There are no shortcuts to physical fitness. You HAVE to put in the work to achieve results. Plain and simple. Energy returned on energy invested. The investment will yield a longer active life.

One of the most overlooked aspects of vitality is your emotional health. Everything from mental health issues like depression and anxiety to disorders like anorexia and schizophrenia can all be linked to an emotional imbalance.

A big part of our conditioning comes from traditional values and culture. Societal conditioning has taught us primitive ways of thinking when it comes to our jobs, circle of friends, family and relationships.

Jobs are supposed to be tough and the road to a successful career is supposed to be strenuous with hills and valleys along the way. Friendships are supposed to be about loyalty and tenure. Family comes first and nothing can or should ever break that bond. Relationships are hard work and happiness is a benefit, not a requirement.

In order to create a healthy life, you have to remove ALL toxicity from your life. ALL includes the job that you can't stand, the friends you've outgrown, the family members who drain your energy and most of all, the partner who's holding you back.

It goes back to my basic philosophy, *Is this choice for the betterment of me or the detriment of me?*

This applies to EVERY decision you make in your life. These choices aren't always easy, but necessary. You have to look at your body, mind and spirit as one. They all work together in harmony or disfunction to represent the essence of you.

Shortcomings in one area will manifest itself in the others. This is a guarantee.

As I pointed out in the Freeing Your Mind section, society has created a work structure designed to benefit the overall function of a system. The idea of working at a job you can't stand just to survive—or working for 50 years only to enjoy a decade or two of retirement—sounds absolutely ridiculous, yet this is the reality for the average American.

The result? Stress, anxiety, depression, substance abuse, regret, and unfulfillment. Does that sound like a healthy life? Is that for the betterment of you or the detriment of you? If your job doesn't bring you joy or fulfillment, you need to be working on an exit plan immediately. This applies to all aspects of your life.

When you start making healthier choices in your life, you'll start to notice your circle getting smaller. This can be alarming at first, but it becomes extremely enlightening once you start to understand what's happening. We are all energy and operate at a certain frequency. As your frequency changes, so does the world around you.

Friends you've known for years start to show up less frequently. You start to realize that you are truly all you need and instead of looking outside of yourself for fulfillment, you look within. It's such an interesting dynamic because instead of searching for happiness, you attract it. Instead of looking for love from other individuals, you look to share your love.

As I continued on my journey towards a healthier life, a good number of friends dropped off. Not because they didn't like me anymore or I didn't like them necessarily, but our energy didn't mesh. Our interests weren't aligned. Topics of conversation were on completely different sides of the spectrum. When you start making healthier choices and notice this happening, allow it and don't feel like you have to hold on to a life or people that no longer align with the new you. Embrace the new you and celebrate it... because you've opened yourself up to a whole new world of possibilities!

This relates to family as well. Blood is thicker than water, yes... but toxic blood will kill you. If your family isn't in line with your values, do not feel obligated to continue that relationship. In my opinion, we have two families. Our blood family and our soul family. We're connected to our blood family solely by our DNA. We're connected to our soul family energetically.

In my opinion, the second most unhealthy element of society behind the food we eat are toxic relationships. People will change their entire persona for the likes of someone else. We, as a people, are so insecure. We don't know our worth and we don't understand the power we possess.

Going back to the question, *Is the person that I'm sharing my life with... my valuable time and energy with... for the betterment of me... or the detriment of me?*

While relationships can be extremely complex due to children, financials etc... the answer to this question gives you a seamless depiction of what you need to do. A healthy life means a life where you are fulfilled, in-balance and uncompromising when it comes to your character and values. It goes back to my discussion on frequency. We're constantly changing.

"Just as a line drawn on water with a stick will quickly vanish and will not last long; even so is human life like a line drawn on water." – Buddha

Sometimes the person you're with isn't on the same frequency as you. Sometimes their journey is different. And that's okay. If you're looking to make healthier changes in your life and your partner is holding you back or unwilling, you have a conscious choice to make. Never stay in an unhappy, unfulfilling or stagnant relationship. The unrest will manifest itself energetically, mentally and physically.

From a physical health perspective, continuing to adhere to toxicity in your relationships has an extremely detrimental effect on your vitality.

Your adrenal glands are the most abused organs in your body, bar none. The adrenal glands sit on top of your kidneys and produce the major hormones that dictate your overall well-being. They also work in conjunction with the autonomic nervous system, dictating fight or flight, assimilation and producing neurotransmitters that transmit signals throughout the body.

When our emotions are out of whack, or should I say out of balance, the adrenal glands are overworked resulting in mood swings, erratic behavior, cognitive issues and mental illness. So, when you wake up dreading your nine-to-five or stressing yourself out before a family function, know that you are adding extreme burden to your body. This can result in overeating, thyroid issues, kidney issues and cause issues with nutritional utilization.

Making life changing decisions with your diet can be a difficult process. Making life decisions when it comes to your job, family, friends and intimate partner can seem excruciating on the surface, but I promise you, it's a very short-termed feeling. When you put yourself first and make your decisions based on the betterment of *you*, you'll always end up in an advantageous situation.

Remember, we've been conditioned to put everyone before ourselves. Our job comes first. Our kids come first. Our spouse comes first. Our country comes first.

Take a drive and observe society around you. Do you see a society that's built for the betterment of you? Or do you see a society that's been created to break you down physically, emotionally and spiritually?

We are all one. We are all connected.

You becoming the best version of yourself affects us all. By you breaking free and creating a healthier life, it enables you to become the best you. By being the best you, you become a better friend, a better parent, a better employee/employer, a better husband/wife, a better colleague, a better son/daughter which ultimately creates a better world for all of us. That is the ripple effect. We all play a part in the collective consciousness of the world and don't ever undermine your impact.

Congratulations on taking the first steps toward detoxing yourself!

Epilogue: What's Next?

If you've made it this far, first — thank you. This book, *Detox Yourself*, was never meant to be just another "how-to" or a checklist you skim through and then put on the shelf. No, this was your wake-up call. The moment where you said, "Enough." Enough to the noise, the overwhelm, the endless conditioning that's been running your mind and body without your true consent.

Look — every one of us has been intoxicated. Not just by food or drink, but by conditioning, programming, invisible forces that shape what we think, how we feel, and the choices we make daily. This conditioning? It's like a fog that keeps you from seeing your own brilliance and your true potential to heal and thrive.

This book was your first step to breaking free from that fog.

Free Your Mind First

Detoxing your body starts with detoxing your mind. You can't truly heal one without the other. The patterns you've absorbed, the stories you tell yourself about your worth, your habits, your limits — these are often the real toxins. They hold you back. They keep you stuck in cycles that no longer serve you.

That's why this journey begins inside. To free your mind means to question everything you think you know about yourself, your health, your life. It means recognizing the lies that culture, society, and even well-meaning people have fed you. And it means choosing to rewrite those narratives with clarity, purpose, and self-love.

Time for a Self-Audit

This is where many people stop, or they only scratch the surface. But you — you're ready for the deep audit. You're ready to look honestly at every part of your life and ask:

- *What is actually serving me — feeding my growth, my peace, my energy?*
- *What is holding me back — draining me, keeping me small, keeping me sick?*

Start with your diet — the very fuel you put into your body. This is your #1 detox target because every bite, every sip, affects your cells, your energy, and your mind. But don't stop there.

Take a hard look at your career. Does your work ignite your spirit or burn it out? Your relationships — are they supportive, uplifting, and loving? Or are they draining and toxic? Your circle, your family dynamics, even your household environment — these are all part of your ecosystem. They can either nourish your growth or poison your peace.

Elimination

Detoxing is not about perfection. It's about progress. It's about removing one toxin at a time — whether it's processed junk in your diet, toxic people in your circle, or limiting beliefs you've carried for years.

Let yourself move at your own pace. There's no race here. The goal is freedom, clarity, and a vibrant life that feels like *you*. When you clear out what no longer serves you, space opens up for new energy, new opportunities, and a deeper connection with your true self.

What's Next? Deeper Into the E.A.T. Philosophy

This book is just the beginning. In my next book, I'll dive deeper into the dietary and health practices that have transformed my life — the foundation of my **E.A.T. Philosophy**. We'll explore not just what to eat, but how to eat in a way that honors your body's natural terrain and supports your mind and spirit.

You'll get practical, actionable steps for nourishing yourself with real, vibrant food — food that heals rather than harms. You'll learn how to listen to your body's wisdom and how to build lasting habits that go beyond quick fixes or fad diets.

A Glimpse Into Your New Path

Before you go, I want to leave you with a snippet from my eBook "The Natural Reset". This guide is designed to give you a clear, seamless transition into healthier dietary habits and a lifestyle that feels authentic and empowering.

Use it as a compass when things feel overwhelming. Let it remind you that this isn't about restriction or deprivation — it's about honoring yourself and stepping into a life that feels full, vibrant, and free.

Final Thoughts

Remember, detoxing yourself is a revolutionary act of self-love and courage. It means breaking the chains of conditioning and taking back control — your mind, your body, your life. It means saying yes to your potential and no to anything that dims your light.

You have everything you need inside you right now. This book was the spark. Now it's time to fan that flame and walk your path to freedom, health, and true joy.

I'm honored to walk this journey with you.

Peace and love,
— R.L. Malpica

The Natural Reset

Your journey to optimal health starts with the body's innate ability to heal itself. This principle, which lies at the core of the terrain model, aligns perfectly with the essence of transitioning to a more natural lifestyle. The following sections from my *Natural Reset eBook* have been adapted and tailored to further enhance *Detox Yourself* with practical strategies and empowering knowledge.

Caloric Intake: Fueling Your Journey

One of the most common misconceptions when transitioning to a natural diet is underestimating the body's caloric needs. While shifting to a raw, fruit-based regimen naturally lightens the digestive load, it's vital to ensure your body receives adequate fuel for daily activities and long-term health.

Why Caloric Intake Matters

During this transition, you will lose water weight due to the elimination of dehydrating, processed foods from your diet. Each fruit-based meal should aim for around 600 calories. For most people, this adds up to 1,500 to 2,000 calories daily, depending on activity level, body size, and specific needs.

Use tools like Chronometer to track your caloric intake and ensure you're meeting your goals. Monitor your weight closely and adjust as necessary to stay nourished and energized.

Food Combining for Optimal Digestion

Good digestion is the cornerstone of a thriving, disease-free body. Food combining principles are essential to maximize digestion efficiency and prevent fermentation in your gut—a major cause of bloating, discomfort, and subpar nutrient absorption.

The Basics of Fruit Combining

- **Sweet Fruits:** Bananas, dates, and figs combine well with other sweet fruits. Avoid mixing with acidic or sub-acid fruits.
- **Sub-Acid Fruits:** Apples, mangoes, and papayas blend seamlessly with sweet or acidic fruits.
- **Acidic Fruits:** Citrus fruits like oranges and pineapples should not be combined with sweet fruits to avoid fermentation.

Improper combinations can slow digestion and cause fermentation, leading to gas, bloating, and discomfort. Keep it simple: focus on one fruit type per meal or ensure compatible combinations to allow your digestive system to work efficiently.

How the Body Cleans Itself: The Terrain Model in Action

The terrain model emphasizes the body's innate intelligence in cleansing and healing itself when given the right conditions. A primary focus of this lifestyle is energy efficiency: when your body isn't bogged down by heavy, processed foods, it reallocates energy to cleaning and repairing.

House Cleaning: Energy and Detoxification

The transition to a fruit-based diet unlocks your body's natural detox mechanisms. During this phase, your body eliminates stored toxins, cellular waste, and metabolic debris. While detox symptoms like fatigue or skin breakouts may arise, they are signs of deep cleansing—progress, not failure.

By embracing hydration from fruits and eliminating processed foods, you free up digestive energy to detoxify and repair tissues, enabling sustained weight loss, better digestion, and renewed vitality.

Building a Lifestyle of Vitality: Weight Loss, Healing, and Beyond

These changes go beyond just weight loss or dietary changes; it's about embracing a holistic shift that touches every aspect of your life. By aligning with the body's natural rhythms and nourishing yourself with nature's foods, you're setting the stage for:

- **Sustainable Weight Loss:** Not through deprivation, but by providing the body with hydrating, nutrient-dense foods.
- **Removing Dis-Ease:** Allowing the body to eliminate inflammation, toxins, and imbalances that contribute to chronic conditions.
- **Emotional and Physical Well-Being:** By reducing toxic influences—whether they're foods, relationships, jobs, or other stressors—you create space for true health and happiness.

Your Tools for Success

This journey isn't just about what you eat; it's about how you live. Below are practical tools to help you along the way:

- **Track Your Progress:** Apps like Chronometer can help ensure you're meeting caloric and nutritional needs.

- **Simplify Meals:** Focus on mono meals or simple combinations to optimize digestion. Start by replacing one full cooked meal a day with raw fruits. Ensure you are eating enough fruit to compensate for the calories of the cooked meal.
- **Stay Patient:** Detox symptoms can be challenging, but they're temporary. Trust your body's process.
- **Seek Support:** Whether through my YouTube channel, personal coaching, or online community, remember you're not alone.

If you're ready to start your transition towards a healthier diet and lifestyle, my eBook "The Natural Reset: A Beginner's Guide to a Transforming Your Health" is available on my website. The guide provides you a pathway to changing your dietary habits and includes an 8-week transition program to help you get on the path to a healthier life! The best time and place to start is right now!

A Note of Gratitude

If you've made it to this page, thank you. Thank you for taking the time to read *Detox Yourself* and for being open enough to challenge your conditioning, question what you've been taught, and take the first steps toward creating a healthier life.

This book isn't just about food or health — it's about freedom. It's about waking up to the systems, beliefs, and influences that don't serve us, and learning how to step into our power with clarity and intention. My deepest hope is that these words planted a seed for you — a seed that will continue to grow long after you put this book down.

If *Detox Yourself* has resonated with you, inspired you, or helped you see things in a new light, I would be truly grateful if you shared your thoughts in an Amazon review. Reviews aren't just about numbers — they're how this message reaches more people who are searching for answers but don't yet know where to turn. Every single review helps amplify the truth and expand this community of people committed to freeing their minds and creating real health.

Your voice matters. Your story matters. And your review could be the reason someone else takes the leap to start their own journey.

With gratitude,
R.L. Malpica